THE EXPECTANT FATHER'S ACTIVITY BOOK

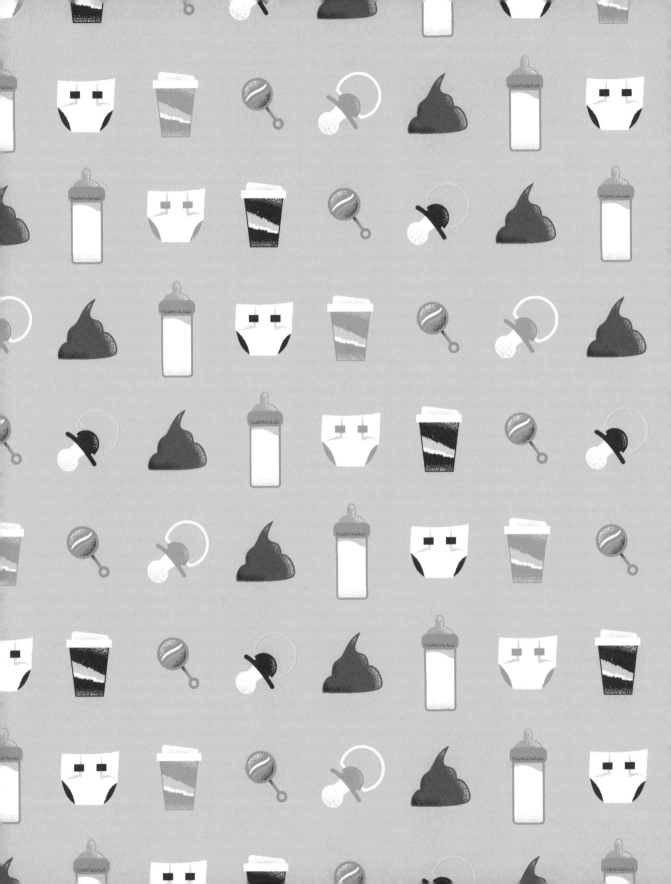

THE EXPECTANT FATHER'S ACTIVITY BOOK

85
Fun Games and Puzzles to Prepare for Fatherhood

James Guttman

ROCKRIDGE PRESS

For Olivia and Lucas, who are the whole reason
I am a proud father today. And for Buddy
and Tipsy, the cats that prepared me for it all.

Interior and Cover Designer: Sean Doyle
Art Producer: Sara Feinstein
Editor: Mo Mozuch
Illustrations © 2020 James Olstein. Art used under license from iStock.com, p. 11.

ISBN: Print 978-1-64739-750-0 | eBook 978-1-64739-451-6
R0

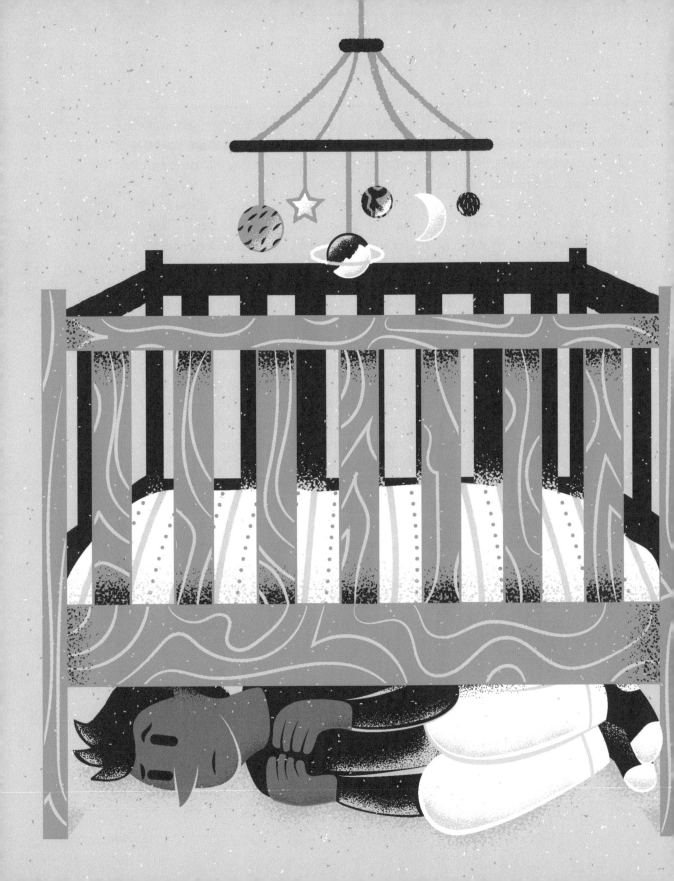

are capable of. For many of us, it's a chance to soar higher than we ever dreamed possible. Self-doubt is normal, but self-actualization is on the horizon. Your child needs you, and the society that they will be a part of one day needs you, too.

You are the moral compass. You are the voice of reason. You're the teller of cautionary tales. Your life, up until this point, has been a learning experience. Your life, going forward, will be a teaching experience. You can use all the tricks you have gathered to help your son or daughter navigate the world before them. All your past mistakes, confusing as they may have been at the time, now have meaning. They all occurred to create lessons for you to one day share with someone else. They all molded you into the teacher you are about to become.

It's a serious subject, but it doesn't have to be overwhelming. Hopefully, this book will provide you with the insight into that delicate balance between knowledge and humor. You can recognize the importance of the lessons while still celebrating the fun of it all. Fatherhood is the ultimate paradox. It's a life or death issue presented with a kid-friendly backdrop. You never know what is around the corner.

So, stick it out, push forward, and do the right thing. The path is hard, but the reward is greater than anything you'll ever experience. It won't be long before you're staring into the eyes of another human being who sees you as a beacon of perfection, and you're left wondering how you ever became so lucky. You'll be amazed at what you can accomplish when the most important person in your world sees you as the most important man in theirs.

You might not get it just yet. But you will. You'll see, Daddy.

Introduction

"Hey, Daddy!"

Like hearing that? You'd better, because everyone is going to say that to you. Everyone . . . on Earth . . . will call you "Daddy."

Relatives will say *"Hey, Daddy. Getting sleep?"*

Waitresses will say *". . . and what will Daddy be having?"*

Like it or not, Daddy will be your new name. When people see a baby, they say it. It's like word association for them. The man with a baby has no name. He's just "daddy." People call the moms "mama," but that transition is easier because women seem to always call each other "mama." Sometimes it seems like none of them know each other's names.

The only ones who won't be calling you "daddy" will be your guy friends. Don't worry. They'll still be calling you "%#&*^&" and "*&%#@!" You may need better friends, but in the meantime, the abusive nicknames will be a welcome change.

But being a daddy and being a father are two very different things. Fathering a child happens only once, at the start of the journey. It takes a single action, and nothing takes that away from you. You carry that honor with you for the rest of your children's lives. Anyone on Earth, no matter who raised them, can say that there is a man out there who is their *father*. For your child, you will be that man. If you are reading this, you have already accomplished that part.

Not everyone can say they have a dad or a daddy. That's more difficult. It's an honor you have to earn and one that you continuously have to renew your rights to throughout life. It's a moniker that comes with offering advice, wisdom, compassion, and love. A daddy is a figure that everyone needs, but not everyone is lucky enough to have. What you do going forward will be what makes you that figure.

Now is your chance to be that light in your children's world. You can offer your next generation a feeling of belonging in a life that can sometimes feel desolate and lonely. It won't be easy. Saying it would, would be a lie. You will have moments where you feel like you've failed and moments where you feel like you want to fail. But, hopefully, a voice inside you will push you to be the best you can be. This is the time to see all you

Contents

PART ONE

Third-to-Last Trimester (Weeks 1–13)

So . . . ready to be a dad? Probably not. You don't feel ready, right? No one does. That's the big secret.

You will never truly feel ready for this. And, if you ever do, that's when life will slap you across the face. Even as you are completing your journey, you'll still feel uneasy about being allowed to bring a baby home. So, rest assured, the first few weeks of expectant fatherhood may feel like imposter syndrome. You might expect men in big coats to come and carry you away in the night so that the real adult can jump in to take your place. You can probably even picture the scene and hear your own scream echoing through the bedroom.

Nope. You're the adult. This is not a drill. This is reality.

Fatherhood is on-the-job training. You're still on probation. Find your desk. Get some coffee. Put on your name tag and sharpen some pencils. You have nine months to learn the massive handbook that is Parenting 101. Don't worry, though. If you don't manage to, you'll have a lifetime to play catch up.

You Got This: Checklist of Things to Hide before the Baby Comes

First things first: you need to see your life through the eyes of a baby. A baby that wants to grab, tug, climb, shake, taste, and swallow everything in sight. Here's a handy list of some household hazards you're probably ignoring because you haven't tried to stick them in your ear . . . yet.

☐ **Drugs:** Over the counter, under the counter, behind the counter. No matter the counter, any medication should be locked away.

☐ **Anything smaller than a block:** If it can block a baby's throat, it shouldn't be anywhere below five feet off the floor. That includes marbles, pennies, candy, nails, and all those things that a wandering bundle of joy might mistake for a snack.

☐ **Weapons:** Both intentional (guns) and creative (spiked shish kebab sticks)

☐ **Alcohol:** Scotch, whisky, bourbon, rubbing

☐ **Household poisons:** Rubbing alcohol is one thing, but any household cleaner typically kept under the sink needs to be locked up or hidden away. Even if a baby can't get into it, a spill of bleach or Lysol on the floor can easily become something that goes into their hands, then their mouths, and then to the hospital.

☐ **Scissors:** You will immediately forget both the hiding place for and your sudden daily need for them, so you buy more, resulting in 10 pairs of scissors hidden throughout your home like a Freddy Krueger Easter egg hunt.

☐ **The good snacks:** Especially the spicy ones

☐ **Plastic bags, or anything like them:** Whether garbage bags, zip-top bags, or even a balloon, it takes nothing for a baby, still struggling with neck strength, to get one pushed against their mouth. Once you start looking around your house, you'll be surprised at how many smothering hazards there actually are.

☐ **The remote control:** Not on purpose, repeat this process every day for the rest of your life.

☐ **Anything you don't want poop on:** Especially the spicy ones

Baby Facts: First Try, Mister

Okay, so maybe you don't know *everything.* This quiz is designed to make you realize that there are lots of things you *do* know. By the end of it, you should feel better about yourself. Score low and, well, you should rethink some things in life.

1. **True or False: Human babies can fly.**
   a) True
   b) False
   c) Depends on the baby

2. **Which of the following is a realistic weight for a newborn baby?**
   a) 5 pounds, 4 ounces
   b) Solid two hundo
   c) Microwave popcorn

3. **How often should you feed your baby?**
   a) Multiple times per day
   b) When they ask you
   c) Trick question; your nipples don't make milk

4. **True or False: Babies wear diapers.**
   a) True
   b) False
   c) Only on Christmas

5. **When do you celebrate your baby's first birthday?**
   a) On the one-year anniversary of baby's birth
   b) Cinco de Mayo, baby!
   c) Babies don't have birthdays. They have dance contests.

6. **Which of the following usually occurs first: crawling, walking, or running?**
   a) Walking
   b) Crawling
   c) Running
   d) All at once

7. **A good choice for a babysitter is:**
   a) A friend or relative you trust
   b) Anyone from Craigslist
   c) Microwave popcorn

Old Wives'/New Moms' Tales

There are things called "old wives' tales." If married, don't make a joke about it to your wife. She won't laugh. These urban legends have long been said to predict a baby's sex. Unscramble the words to these myths and look smart when sharing useless trivia with your in-laws. What a fun life you have now!

If the baby bump looks like a absbaktlel __ __ __ __ __ __ __ __ __ __, it's a boy. It

also might just be a absbaktlel __ __ __ __ __ __ __ __ __ __. That would be sweet.

A twese ohtto __ __ __ __ __ __ __ __ __ __ is a sign that the baby may be a girl,

while aytsl vrigacsn __ __ __ __ __ __ __ __ __ __ __ __ are signs for a boy.

Most men reading this now think they are pregnant with twins.

Boys give pregnant moms locd tefe __ __ __ __ __ __ __ __.

Selunmicss __ __ __ __ __ __ __ __ __ __ means it's a boy. Of course, they call it an

old *wives'* tale. So, it sounds like something that a man wouldn't have written.

If her right streab __ __ __ __ __ __ is larger during pregnancy, it's a boy. A larger left

is a girl. If the middle one is largest, that means you probably got a Martian pregnant.

Wogglin inks __ __ __ __ __ __ __ __ __ __ __ is the sign of a boy. Then again, so

is radiation poisoning.

Lenwols slekan __ __ __ __ __ __ __ __ __ __ __ __ __ are usually a sign for boys.

Grithb epe __ __ __ __ __ __ __ __ __ is the sign of a boy. If not, it's a girl. Think of

a little yellow cup wearing a graduation cap.

Boys are said to add half a hose seiz __ __ __ __ __ __ __ __ to mothers.

Glanilf paesle __ __ __ __ __ __ __ __ __ __ __ __ __ on your right side is a sign

of a girl. Because girls are always right, right? See?

Girls give the moms baruhnetr __ __ __ __ __ __ __ __ __. In 13 years, dads will

get it, too.

Grontser snail __ __ __ __ __ __ __ __ __ __ __ __ __ are signs of a boy. Freddy

Krueger is having a boy.

Grontser raih __ __ __ __ __ __ __ __ __ __ __ __ is, too. Throws the Freddy

theory out the window.

Paging Doctor Google: Colic

You know what colic is?
Oh, good.

Wait. Do you think it is part of your hairline? No. That's not it. You don't know. Glad we clarified that.

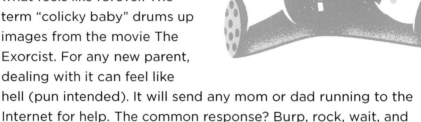

Colic is stomach pain that some babies suffer from, and it causes them to cry for what feels like forever. The term "colicky baby" drums up images from the movie The Exorcist. For any new parent, dealing with it can feel like hell (pun intended). It will send any mom or dad running to the Internet for help. The common response? Burp, rock, wait, and hope. This too shall pass.

One of the most Googled terms for babies is RSV, otherwise known as Respiratory Syncytial Virus. Although it can affect anyone, babies are most susceptible due to their underdeveloped nasal passages. It makes it much harder for them to get mucus out of their tiny heads. The most common treatment is a bulb, similar to a turkey baster, which sucks the boogies from their little noses. Check with your doctor, and don't panic. Never panic.

You may want to panic, though, when you first notice that your baby came home with the cord that originally plugged them into their mother like a toaster oven. To save you the question and web search, it's called an umbilical cord and not an "oh my God, I'm gonna throw up." It falls off a week or two after birth, leaving a belly button behind. I suggest that you try not to mention it . . . or look in that general direction.

They Named Them What?!

Celebrities name their babies some weird names. No, it's not the start of a "Who's on First" skit. It's the start of a crossword puzzle. The name of the celeb is provided. You need to determine what they named that poor kid . . .

ACROSS

1. Things were looking up for Kanye and Kim Kardashian West.

3. Sting and Frances Tomelty were tickled pink upon the birth of their baby.

6. Steven Spielberg and Kate Capshaw were slinging more than guns when they named this baby, partner.

8. Chris Martin and Gwyneth Paltrow were looking to keep any doctors away from their baby.

9. Jim Toth and Reese Witherspoon were in a state of Graceland when their baby arrived.

10. Forest Whitaker and Keisha Nash Whitaker really named their kid this. Honest. No lie.

11. Brad Pitt and Angelina Jolie Pitt were years before their own personal civil war battle when they had her.

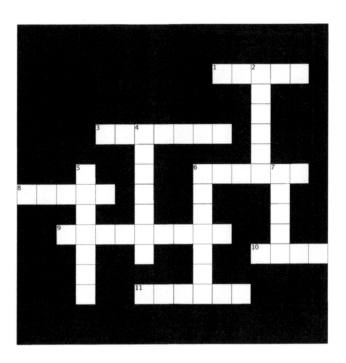

DOWN

2. Robert Rodriguez and Elizabeth Avellán soared to new heights with this name, man.

4. Marc Silverstein and Busy Philipps bowled this one out of the field.

5. Jay-Z and Beyoncé made sure to leave a lasting hue with this one.

6. Dpop goes Frank Zappa and Adelaide Gail Zappa's dbaby.

7. Bruce Willis and Demi Moore spilled some tea when they named this one.

Father of the Remote Control:
EUGENE POLLEY

The next time you change channels during the commercial without having to get up and kneel, you might want to drop to a knee anyway and thank Eugene Polley. In 1955, Polley invented the first ever remote control. Under the snazzy name "Flash-Matic," Polley's clicker was connected by wire and could control volume and power, allowing users to channel flip without getting out of their (presumably asbestos-filled) chairs. In some ways, he may have been the father of the couch potato, too. His work for Zenith also included car radios and video discs, but nothing ever came close to the magic of the remote. It also makes Polley the father of the phrase "Where the hell did I leave the remote control?!"

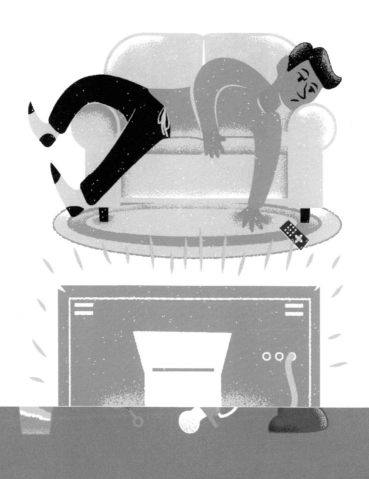

Pot Net Manes

What were the top ten male and female baby names of the 2000s? Unscramble the names to find out. Just pretend you're a substitute teacher, with a hangover, taking attendance.

bajoc — — — — —

melyi — — — — —

helimac — — — — — — —

odanims — — — — — — —

sajhou — — — — — —

aema — — — —

mtwheat — — — — — — —

ivloai — — — — — —

aldnie — — — — — —

nahnah — — — — — —

sorchhtierp — — — — — — — — — — —

bilaiga — — — — — — —

wander — — — — — —

blaseail — — — — — — —

netha — — — — —

tahmansa — — — — — — — —

pesjho — — — — — —

ethabziel — — — — — — — — —

i am lwil — — — — — — —

elshay — — — — — —

Expecting?

ACROSS

2. Something you expect to take an hour, but takes like a whole day.

5. Something you expect to be hot, but is usually cold.

7. Some people you expect to leave, but never do.

8. Something you expect to be blamed for, and will be.

13. Something you are told to do, but will annoy the nurses during delivery.

14. Something you expect to do at some point, but never do.

16. Something you don't expect to smell as bad as it does.

18. Something you expect your partner to do, but never so much.

19. Something you expect to be free, but is expensive.

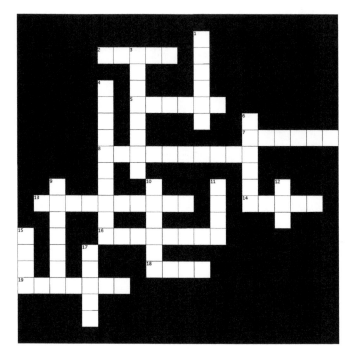

DOWN

1. Someone who is expecting when you show up, but not when you leave.

3. Something you expect to be easy to remove, but isn't.

4. Something you expect to be impossible, but you handle it like a boss.

6. Something you expect to get from the hospital, but don't anymore.

9. Something you expected to pack before, but usually forget.

10. Something you expect to be helpful, but isn't.

11. Something you expect they would never let you leave the hospital with, but they do.

12. Something you are constantly reminded is not allowed for months after.

15. Something you are not prepared to see on the delivery table.

17. Something you are not prepared to see on your new baby.

My Baby Is As Big As . . .

Fruit is boring. Sure it's healthy and delicious, but you're going to get tired of every baby growth chart tracking the journey from poppy seed to pumpkin. Instead, here's a handy guide of much cooler objects so your friends' eyes don't glaze over when you try to talk to them about how big your kickass baby is getting. These are approximate measurements based mostly on length—your baby won't actually look like a DVD player at 32 weeks (relax).

4–7 weeks
Baby starts out about the size of the "like" button and grows to the size of your pinky fingernail.

16–19 weeks
Baby starts out about the size of a twinkie and grows to the size of a dollar bill.

28–31 weeks
Baby starts out about the size of a bowling pin and grows to the size of a large movie theater popcorn.

8–11 weeks
Baby starts out about the size of an app icon on your phone and grows to the size of a beer cap.

20–23 weeks
Baby starts about out the size of a video game controller and grows to the size of a chicken burrito.

32–35 weeks
Baby starts out about the size of a DVD player and grows to the size of a baby boa constrictor.

12–15 weeks
Baby starts out about the size of a golf ball and grows to the size of a cassette tape.

24–27 weeks
Baby starts out about the size of an empty paper towel roll and grows to the size of a wooden spatula.

36–40 weeks
Baby starts out the size of a necktie and grows to the size of your new baby!

Baby Names for Bathroom Terms

Your baby only urinates and makes bowel movements when you talk to the doctor. To friends, family, and the baby themself, it makes all sorts of other things. Search for all the words that describe baby waste. It's kind of gross, yes. But if you think doing this activity is gross, then you're not ready for what you're going to spend the next couple of years wiping up.

Poop	Uh-Oh	Cigar	Sprinkle
Doodie	Piddle	CharlieBrownie	Crapsicle
Doo-Doo	Wee-Wee	Wizz	Snickerdoodle
Caca	Pee-Pee	Leak	
Stinky	Deuce	Squirt	
Yucky	Loaf	Tinkle	

```
T  P  V  E  W  Q  Z  Y  S  T  I  N  K  Y  P
F  O  Y  L  W  E  S  Z  Z  I  W  U  E  R  E
G  O  D  D  E  G  E  A  C  O  N  J  I  A  W
T  P  X  O  H  D  R  W  B  Q  M  J  N  G  S
B  K  Y  O  O  E  E  P  E  E  P  C  W  I  P
I  T  H  D  Y  D  H  K  K  E  I  J  O  C  R
E  U  P  R  K  S  O  I  C  V  D  T  R  L  I
S  F  V  E  C  X  K  O  R  R  D  W  B  H  N
Q  H  K  K  U  L  A  Y  A  A  L  C  E  D  K
U  E  T  C  Y  Z  K  U  P  F  E  W  I  L  L
I  L  L  I  V  B  A  R  S  H  E  L  L  B  E
R  K  X  N  L  M  K  K  I  I  C  E  R  K  T
T  N  M  S  V  O  A  N  C  Z  U  A  A  J  C
E  I  D  O  O  D  A  M  L  D  E  K  H  M  V
O  T  I  V  B  J  M  F  E  Q  D  B  C  Q  P
```

Empathy Exercise

This is the time to be thoughtful. If you've been saving up an idea for an anniversary or special event, this is the special event. In fact, this is the only special event. Your whole life has been leading to this special event. Think of your romantic gestures as a rainy-day fund and these nine months as one long rainy day. Spend your sweet capital. It will be appreciated one thousand-fold. When you combine pregnancy emotions, hormones, and a genuinely important event, it makes for the perfect storm of consideration. Be the thunder rather than the downpour. To quote the movie *Lean on Me*: "Go buy her some stupid gold."

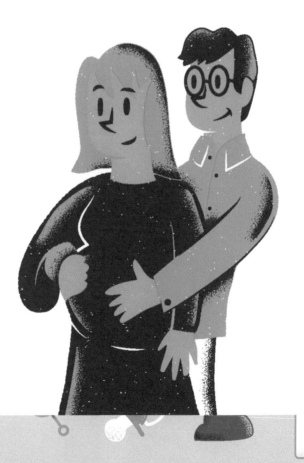

Netflix and Dad

While you still have something that resembles free time, it might be a good idea to brush up on some fatherhood movies. Here's a list of some classics, from feel-goods to feel-scared-to-deaths to just feels, to help you track your "research."

The Funny

☐ *Dutch*

☐ *Mrs. Doubtfire*

☐ *Look Who's Talking*

☐ *Parenthood*

☐ *Three Men and a Baby*

☐ *Big Daddy*

☐ *Uncle Buck*

☐ *Finding Nemo*

The Feels

☐ *Field of Dreams*

☐ *He Got Game*

☐ *My Life*

☐ *Boyz n the Hood*

☐ *Pursuit of Happyness*

☐ *Big Fish*

☐ *The Lion King*

The Frightening

☐ *The Stepfather*

☐ *Rosemary's Baby*

☐ *Freddy's Dead, The Final Nightmare*

☐ *The Shining*

☐ *The Amityville Horror*

☐ *Mrs. Doubtfire* (if you really think about it)

☐ *Oldboy*

Wack Facts

Take a moment to enjoy some weird little tidbits about babies. Some are made up. All, however, are strange.

1. A baby is unable to taste salt until the four-month mark. T / F

2. 92 percent of babies are born with 11 toes, with the extra one falling off after one week. T / F

3. The intestines of a newborn are around 11 feet long. T / F

4. Babies are born without kneecaps. T / F

5. A baby is born with a thin layer of wax around the ears, which is the same kind used to make organic crayons. T / F

6. Babies are born with a natural swimming ability and can hold their breath, but this ability disappears quickly. T / F

7. Some babies are born with teeth in their ears, which fall out within hours after birth. T / F

8. A group of babies is called a "gaggle." T / F

9. A newborn baby has roughly one cup of blood in their entire body. T / F

10. For an entire year, the CEO of Ford Motor Company was a baby, for tax purposes. T / F

11. A newborn baby can kick with the force of a full-grown goose. T / F

12. Babies have more bones than adults. T / F

13. Worldwide, the most common baby name in all of history is "Yoda." T / F

14. Babies may cry, but they don't produce tears. T / F

15. Babies' first poop doesn't smell and looks like tar. T / F

16. Baby hair falls out because it is mostly made up of pee protein. T / F

17. The first baby formulas were made using baby saliva. T / F

18. Babies only see black and white for the first three months. T / F

19. A baby's brain doubles in size over the first year of life. T / F

20. Babies are born with rabies, hence the name. T / F

Author's Advice

Get a battery jumper for your car. Jumper cables? No. Battery jumper. It's basically a portable car battery that you can jump your car within five minutes. The average cost is about $100, making it around the cost of two jumps from roadside assistance. It may be easy to listen to the radio for 30 minutes while a tow truck shows up, or to search for a random motorist to let you attach your cables to their engine. But when a baby is involved, even the easiest of things become difficult. You'll see. Making a cup of coffee with a screaming infant can be a hassle. Imagine trying to get your battery up and running with one. It's a special ring of hell. Be prepared.

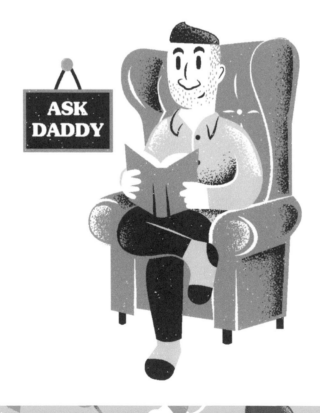

ASK DADDY

I Want My Baby to Grow Up to Be Like (BLANK).

Your child can be anything one day. That sounds like a good thing. Sometimes it is. Sometimes it's not. Use the word bank to match the famous name to their childhood roots.

1. Queen Elizabeth II's cousin describes her as _____.

2. Kim Jong-un's childhood friends say he was shy and _____.

3. According to Marvel Comics, a young Peter Parker, a.k.a. Spiderman, was _____.

4. She is famous for her work with radiation, but as a child, Marie Curie was _____.

5. Believe it or not, a young Tupac Shakur was _____.

6. Before he was the first man on the moon, Neil Armstrong was _____.

7. Football legend Walter Payton was _____ in high school.

8. Friends considered a young Kurt Cobain of Nirvana to be _____ _____.

9. Before his days as "Macho Man," WWE wrestler Randy Savage was _____.

10. Jane Austen was _____ at age eight.

11. Under his father's guidance, Bruce Lee was actually _____.

12. In his early teens, O. J. Simpson was _____.

13. As a boy, Pope John Paul II was _____.

CONTINUED >

I Want My Baby to Grow Up to Be Like (BLANK). CONTINUED

14. Elvis Presley was _____ at the age of 10.

15. Before his infamous "family," Charles Manson was _____.

16. As a girl, Jacqueline Kennedy Onassis was _____.

17. Before shattering gender barriers in tennis, a young Billie Jean King was _____.

18. Although she later became famous for her astronautic pursuits, a young Sally Ride was _____.

19. Unconventional for women at the time, a young Martha Washington was actually _____.

20. At age 16, Joan Rivers was _____.

in a street gang	a softball player
a talented cartoonist	an Eagle Scout
a ballerina	vice president of the Dramatic Club
a minor league baseball player	a jolly girl
a horse stable boy	the second-place winner of a
bullied	youth talent show
a marching band drummer	a gold-medal recipient in gym
a tennis player	a basketball fan
a Shakespearean actor	an avid reader
deathly ill	a soccer goalkeeper
a child actor	

The Poop Scoop

In the first year, the average baby has 2,300 diaper changes. That means if you allowed every major league baseball player at the start of the season to change one diaper, each would get three turns at the pee-pee plate. Batter up.

If you found diapers on the black market for 25 cents each, you'd still spend close to $600 on them in the first year. Thinking that's *"full of *%#"*? You're right. But it's still true.

The word "diaper" in the USA is from a term for "ornamental cloth." The term "nappy" in Britain comes from "napkin." Neither of them seems to fit, since you would never wear one as an ornamental cloth or wipe your mouth with one after eating hot wings.

Marion Donovan is credited for creating disposable diapers when she introduced the world to "boaters" in 1946. These were plastic covers for cloth diapers. Her original prototype was made from disposable shower curtains, which, if you've ever been urinated on by a baby, makes total sense.

In 1982, 43 percent of fathers said they had never changed a diaper. By 2000, it was only 3 percent who made that claim. So, get ready to change some diapers. The days of smoking a pipe outside the delivery room and enlisting in World War II are over.

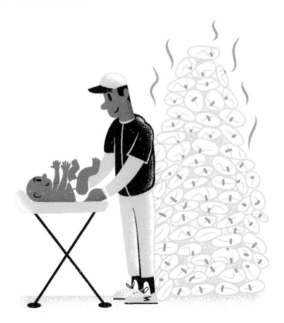

Dad Jokes Lighter (Like a Match, only Better)

Hey, you know Dad jokes? Well, he does. Dad tells jokes. See how it works? Match the words to the appropriate eye-rolling response. Why twice? Because the first 'sponse wasn't enough. Getting it yet?

1. Neck Tie
2. Watch Cartoons
3. Rubber Band
4. Juice Box
5. iPhone
6. Road Trip
7. Ice Cream Sundae

8. Milkshake
9. Nursery School
10. Mail Man
11. Nursery Rhyme
12. Toilet Paper
13. Toilet Bowl
14. High Chair

15. Fast Food
16. Doctor's Bill
17. Nintendo
18. Bread Sticks
19. Baby Formula
20. Diaper Change

_____ Hello, table!

_____ I prefer rock music, but that sounds like it has some bounce to it.

_____ I'd rather have beer money.

_____ After that, we're sending her to Doctery School.

_____ Easy. One part mom. One part dad. Two parts poop.

_____ Is that when two throats score the same amount of points?

_____ Maybe you spilled glue on it.

_____ I could only listen, especially if I was the one driving.

_____ Ninten-Doh!

_____ I read it, but the headlines are all about poop.

_____ Must have been one scared cow.

_____ I didn't know he was a duck.

_____ I also fax.

_____ How will we ever catch it?

_____ That name is kind of redundant.

_____ Why would Juice want to fight anyone?

_____ How? It can't roll a ball!

_____ She should have tied her shoelaces.

_____ Uh . . . Bursery, mursery, cursery.

_____ You do? I yell every day.

Things to Never Say to Your Pregnant Partner . . . or Should You?

Answer True or False to the following statements: True if you should say them to your pregnant partner and false if not. The alternative is to just try them all out and see which ones get you violently attacked. Our way is safer.

1. Wow. It's like you're glowing.
   T / F

2. Whoa. Slow down, killer. Save some ice cream for the rest of us. T / F

3. I can't wait to be a daddy! T / F

4. My feet hurt. T / F

5. I bet I could have a baby. T / F

6. I would love to see pictures from your baby shower again. T / F

7. Does Uber go to the hospital? T / F

8. Can I get you something to eat or drink? A pillow for your head, perhaps? T / F

9. I bet I could fit that maternity shirt around the couch. T / F

10. It's so sweet that your mother is offering to stay with us. She will be a big help! T / F

11. Ugh. I'm not sure I can take nine months of this. T / F

12. We're going to be such great parents! T / F

13. Do stretch marks go away?
    T / F

14. No. That food combination isn't weird at all. You're not weird at all. You're perfect. T / F

15. Your shoelaces are untied. Oh wait . . . can you not see your feet? T / F

16. I'm counting down the days!
    T / F

17. I'm not suggesting it because it's my ex-girlfriend's name. I'm suggesting it because it's a nice name for a baby! T / F

Kiss That Life Goodbye

What are you going to miss about your old life? Well, unscramble these words and you'll know. Actually, you don't need to unscramble them. You'll know soon enough.

nakdryud — — — — — — — —

lets plaee — — — — — — — — —

trap widly — — — — — — — — —

seencil — — — — — — —

cayvirp — — — — — — —

legp oitiklns menele — — — — — — — — — — — —

goutigon — — — — — — — —

eymon — — — — —

sixeetmy — — — — — — — —

omivont — — — — — — —

shwim — — — — —

colors ac — — — — — — — —

story delch — — — — — — — — — —

dis danghtut — — — — — — — — — — —

josi wrasdnn — — — — — — — — — —

disngepe — — — — — — — —

ruscnig — — — — — — —

snief dyseder — — — — — — — — — — — —

elantimeo — — — — — — — — —

pluse thleglnife — — — — — — — — — — — — —

bisstreriiinopyl — — — — — — — — — — — — — —

In This Trimester

This is the trimester where you meet your partner's OBGYN. Prepare to bring your partner to appointments, endure long waits, and remember said appointments. If only there were some kind of hilarious dad activity book to entertain you
. . . hmm.

Ultrasound pictures are difficult to make out, even when the baby is the size of a watermelon. Until then, it's damn near impossible. Learn to pretend. When they point to a blob of black and white swirls and say, *"This is the head,"* nod as if to say, *"Yes. Head. I have heard of heads."*

The heartbeat is far easier to make out. For dads lost at the OBGYN, hearing the baby's heartbeat for the first time is unforgettable. All snark and *"I don't know what I'm doing"* daddy stuff aside, it's a memorable moment. Embrace and remember it.

You will be eager to help your partner in this early stage, but pace yourself. You have nine months. If she insists that she can still get up and get the remote, let her. Don't make her feel helpless. The thought that she may have to let you do every single thing for nine months might be enough to send an able-bodied woman over the edge.

Who's Your Baby?

Take the following parenting instructions and then search for the type of person your child will be, based on your actions. It says as much about you as them.

Praise school, learning, and respect for teachers

Encourage laughter and jokes around the house

Teach empathy

Slip candy and cigarettes into their pockets at convenience stores and tell them, *"It's okay, big companies can afford it"*

Tell them the monsters under their bed are real . . . and hungry

Shave their head in a Mohawk and give them gold chains to help them pity the fools

Tell them that the TV watches them sleep at night and reports to the government

Make them practice sports constantly

Put little bowties on their diapers

A	B	Y	P	A	R	A	N	O	I	D	K	E	Z	R
Q	K	X	I	J	A	C	K	E	D	N	O	L	E	A
U	Q	X	I	Y	W	C	J	S	H	I	X	P	W	C
I	S	Q	D	C	Z	N	Y	P	W	Q	P	S	L	R
I	D	K	V	G	E	A	K	N	I	A	M	J	B	I
W	J	S	E	U	E	U	V	N	D	A	M	M	X	M
R	E	H	T	O	R	B	O	I	R	A	M	R	Q	I
D	R	C	S	F	Z	C	X	T	O	Y	P	S	T	N
F	I	Z	Y	D	E	I	F	I	R	R	E	T	E	A
P	W	N	U	N	N	I	L	M	E	R	G	K	L	L
D	R	Y	H	P	N	S	P	H	D	A	I	Y	O	U
O	K	P	L	I	Y	U	Q	P	E	N	L	R	N	H
C	C	P	T	Z	E	M	F	E	D	N	C	A	H	K
P	P	U	S	Z	D	E	T	S	U	A	H	X	E	P
U	Z	P	R	A	X	B	A	T	M	A	N	I	Q	V

Don't feed them after midnight

Show them how to jump on turtles, find coins in bricks

Cover in cheese and sauce

Hang crib upside down

Lift!

Teach to fetch slippers and hate mailman

The Ultimate Goal— without the bad parts

Empathy Exercise

Joking about how big a pregnant woman is fine for sitcoms, but it is bad for life. You may think, *"It's funny because it's true,"* but she will surely think it's not funny because it's true. Before you try to defend your witty banter with personal experiences, know that it's not alike. In this case, you're essentially laughing at the life you both created. It may sound extreme, but that's how she sees it because, well, that's how it is. Think about it. So, ease up, Seinfeld. She's not going to laugh along or "take a joke." Your humor is better used on other subjects like flatulence and puns.

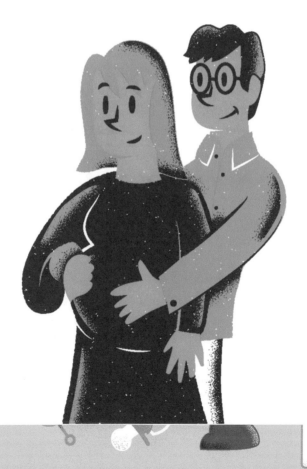

Who Will I Be?

The type of dad you are is ultimately up to you. But first, you need to know what type of dads there are. Match the type of dad to the description.

1. Clueless Dad
2. Grumpy Dad
3. Sports Dad
4. Funny Dad
5. Cool Dad
6. "In My Day" Dad
7. Old Dad
8. Army Dad

_____ Dad who thinks he's hilarious. No one else really does, but they're polite to him about it . . . usually.

_____ Uses militant language to "get things shipshape." Most susceptible to receiving rude faces and hand gestures when back is turned.

_____ Doesn't know where to find the peanut butter. Says "Ask your mother" for every question, including "How are you doing?"

_____ To a kid, any of us. All of us.

_____ Speaks in grumbly sighs and pained expressions.

_____ Tries to use language popular among the younger crowd. Uses it wrong. Puts "the" in front of everything (the Instagram, the Twitter, etc.).

_____ Calls kids "slugger" and "champ." Talks about throwing around the ol' (whatever ball is available).

_____ Has a story about everything that goes back to "his day."

A Never-Google List

Never Google *"Why is my baby turning (color)?"* No matter what color you are about to write, don't Google. Go to the hospital. The only color a baby should be is baby color.

Never Google *"What is wrong with my baby's (body part)?"* No matter what body part you put in, you are going to see some horrendous stuff in the Images section. Medieval horror shows. Be more specific. Or go to the hospital.

Never Google *"Could (BLANK) kill a baby?"* Even if you are innocently making sure something is safe, that looks bad on your search history. Plus, if you have to Google it, then yes. Probably it will. Seriously. I shouldn't have to tell you this. You're gonna be a dad. Use your head.

Empathy Exercise

Be enthusiastic, but let her vent. You may be tired, but she's more tired. You may be moody, but she's moodier. If you're having a good day and she's not, let her get it out. The more you relate, the happier she'll be. No one wants a lecture when they're growing another person inside them. If you don't know what "mansplaining" is, this is the time when you get it 'splained to you. Just remember one simple thing. If she's mad about something, let her tell you all about it and be glad it's not *you* she's mad at. Try to convince her she's "oversensitive," and she won't be complaining to you, she'll be complaining *about* you. That's how you end up getting nicknames from her girlfriends.

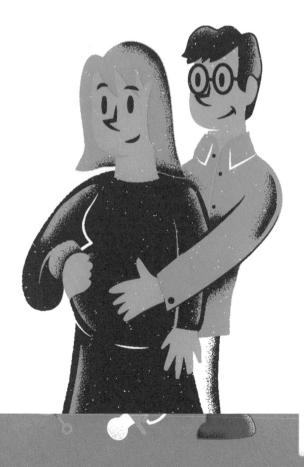

"Bad" Dad Jokes vs. "Bad Dad" Jokes

Everyone loves a good dad joke. Funnily enough, everyone loves a bad dad joke too. The only caveat is that they should be told by a good dad. What's the difference between a "bad" dad joke and a "bad dad" joke? It's more than quote placement. See if you can tell the difference and circle the one that fits your bad dad style.

1. **Make me a milkshake.**

   Poof! You're a milkshake.

   You don't deserve a milkshake. You're a disappointment as a child.

2. **I'm hungry.**

   Hi, hungry. I'm Dad!

   That's because I spent all of our food money at the track.

3. **Dad: I got us a new dog without a nose. Do you know how he smells?
   Kid: How?**

   Awful!

   He doesn't. Our dog has no nose. I got him on a discount. He also has a contagious disease. Don't pet him. I think it's rickets.

4. **What time is my dentist appointment?**

   Tooth hurty!

   We're just going to have the barber look at your teeth. He charges less.

5. **We're driving past a cemetery.**

   People are dying to get in there.

   We'll all be there. Soon. All of us. Life is a void. A dark, eternal void. All your pets will die. All your friends will die. You . . . you will die. Happy Birthday.

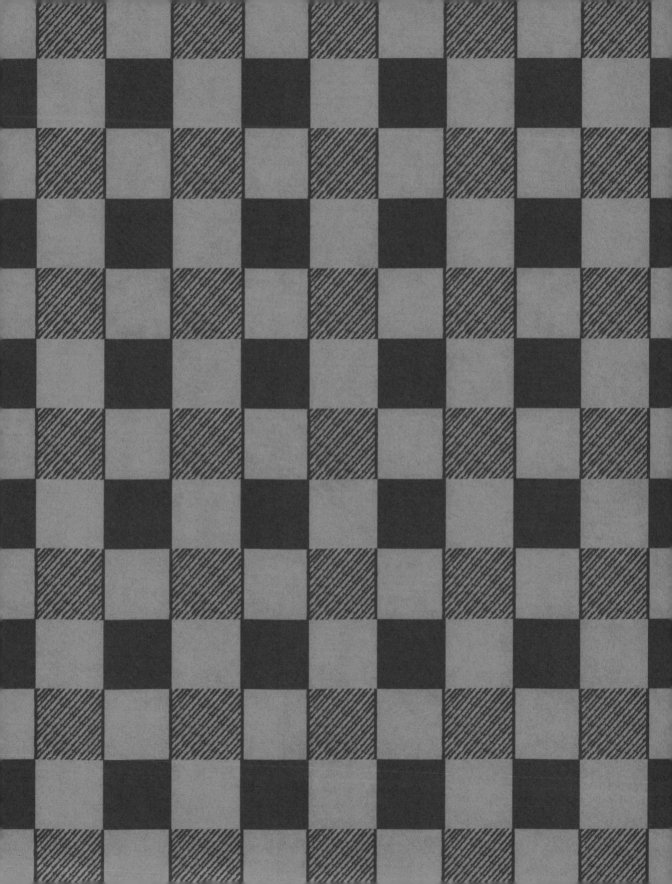

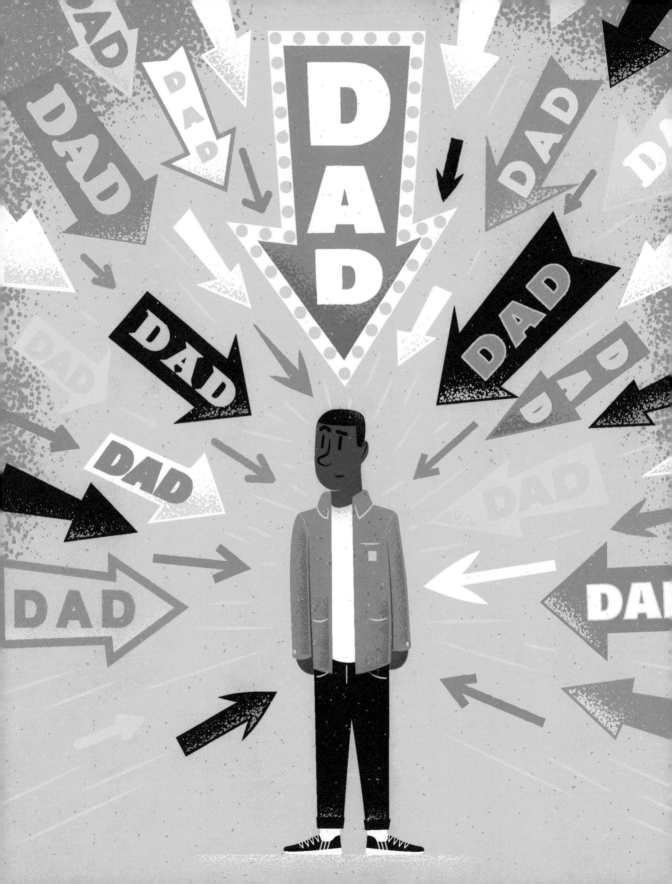

PART TWO

Second-to-Last Trimester (Weeks 14–27)

You made it! Welcome to the Second Trimester Club.

This is the part of the pregnancy journey when things start to feel "real." The initial shock of *Wow, is this really happening?* has (mostly) subsided, and now it's time to tell the world. Once you make it past about three months, the news begins to get shared with family, friends, and neighbors. It's no longer your little secret. It's out for everyone to know.

You may feel more nervous now than you did before, which is totally normal. It's all a trial by fire, and as you move forward, the information is going to come at you fast and furious. Just absorb what you can and hold on. It will all be worth it. No dads-to-be feel like they fully "get it" yet. That just means that you want to do the best you can do, and that's commendable.

So, pat yourself on the back. Maybe have a beer to toast yourself. Just, you know, don't let her see you. She'll get jealous because she can't have one. Maybe have two, then. One for you and one for her. Wouldn't want to let a good beer go to waste.

Second Try, Mister

Time is moving on, and you're getting more adept at this expectant dad thing? OK. Let's up the ante and make things a bit tougher. Choose the best answer to each question. No pressure. This is only . . . the rest of your life! AH!

1. **What is Braxton Hicks?**
   a) False labor pains
   b) Real labor pains
   c) That dipstick who sold you that bum Toyota
   d) Rednecks who live in Braxton

2. **In this trimester, it is helpful to watch the following kinds of videos online:**
   a) Childbirth videos
   b) Japanese Deathmatch Wrestling
   c) People playing video games
   d) Cats doing cute cat things

3. **What should a woman NOT take for a headache during this time period?**
   a) Aspirin
   b) Lemon Pledge
   c) A chill pill
   d) All of the above

4. **What does OBGYN stand for?**
   a) Obstetrician Gynecologist
   b) Oh boy! Getting yummy noodles!
   c) Orange banana grape yogurt Nestea
   d) Truth, Justice, and the American Way

5. **At this stage of pregnancy, a baby's digestive system is fully formed. This means that they can:**
   a) Taste food
   b) Spit mad rhymes
   c) Make gagging noises when listening to your crappy CDs
   d) Move out and get a job

6. **At 26 weeks, babies are able to:**
   a) Beatbox
   b) Dab
   c) Blink their eyes
   d) Blink someone else's eyes . . . using their minds

7. **You should call the doctor if a pregnant woman experiences any of the following except:**
   a) Jaundice
   b) Vomiting
   c) Nausea
   d) Happiness

8. **At this stage, babies in the womb develop a thin coat of wax over their skin, which is disgustingly referred to as:**
   a) Cheesy Varnish
   b) Castrol GTX
   c) Soul Glo
   d) Nasty!

9. **A procedure where a doctor removes a small amount of fluid from the uterus to test a baby's lung capacity is called:**
   a) An amniocentesis
   b) Auntie old sent thesis
   c) "In Utero" by Nirvana
   d) Tappin' the ol' keg

10. **At this point, you can typically find out your baby's:**
    a) Preferred sports team
    b) Credit score
    c) Favorite Adam Sandler movie
    d) Sex

11. **At this stage of pregnancy, couples are encouraged to do what with their birth hospital?**
    a) Sue them
    b) Call it the Drop Zone
    c) Spray paint "baby time" on the parking garage wall
    d) Take a tour

Crossing Words and Changing Bodies

Your partner is changing. Have you noticed? This crossword puzzle will get you up to speed.

ACROSS

2. Braxton Hicks is another term for false . . .

5. Low blood pressure can cause this in pregnant women.

6. These usually appear during the second trimester, meaning you are no longer the only pain in/on your pregnant partner's butt.

7. A problem you might get from chewing glass, something that comes with vampire baseball cards, and a problem that women typically face in the second trimester.

10. Three-letter abbreviation of something you should learn at this stage.

11. Pelvic exercises women do to prepare for the baby. Sounds like something you eat with kreame kheese.

13. Another term for the, ugh, answer for 5 across is varicose.

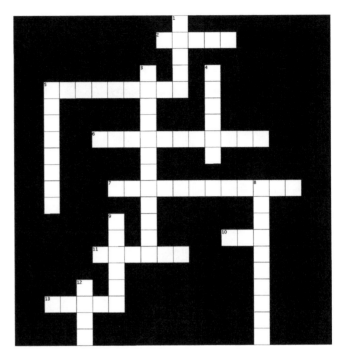

DOWN

1. Besides ankles and breasts, women typically see these body parts swell during pregnancy. High five!

3. This typically drops in males during their partner's pregnancy.

4. Shockingly, a female newborn might get this once or twice after birth. It feels like I should have an exclamation point here, but no. It's something else.

5. Pregnant moms are usually tested for this Wilford Brimley disease through a blood test.

8. Snapshot inside the stomach for your baby's first doctor-assisted selfie.

9. This typically expands inside of a woman during the second trimester.

12. At this stage, you can actually feel your little Bruce Lee do this.

Author's Advice

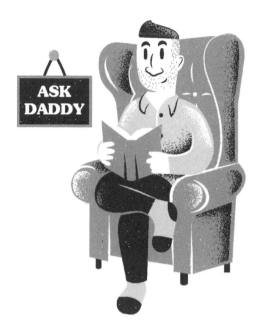

ASK DADDY

At this point, you're probably narrowing down a name for your little bundle of joy. Regardless of its sex, you're good to go. It took work, research, and compromise. You're probably really proud of yourselves, huh? Naming a baby is no joke. You can't just pick a TV character and tack it on like you did with the dog, right? Aw, isn't that right, little Mr. Gitty Goomba? Woofy, woofy, woomba. Who's a good boy? You're a good boy. Yes, you are. Aw.

Here's some free advice: tell no one. No matter how great you think the name is or how much you are sure they will love it, don't utter a word. The last thing you need is a story about how *"I once knew a Drew who tried to shoot my father"* or an upturned eyebrow from Grandma with a snide *"Surely you can't be serious."*

It will haunt you forever. If need be, think of a terrible fake name to throw out as a decoy. Tell them it's Reximillian or something. Watch the looks of disgust and then imagine that look as a response to the real name you plan on using. Doesn't feel so good, right? You're welcome.

That's a Terrible Name There, Sparky

How do you feel about your choice for a baby name? Happy? You do? Oh wait, that's the name? Happy? Oh. Okay. That's great. Anyway . . . it's not as bad as it could have been. Read the following list and check the ones that are actual baby names found in U.S. census records. The answer will shock you, Happy.

1. Arse (FL, 1898) T / F
2. Drug (AL, 1848) T / F
3. Lasagna (NC, 1968) T / F
4. Gassy (SC, 1888) T / F
5. Flappy (KY, 1994) T / F
6. Justin Case (NY, 1832) T / F
7. Sucker (NC, 1896) T / F
8. Poof (IA, 1859) T / F
9. Spicy (GA, 1859) T / F
10. R. U. Ready (KS, 1896) T / F
11. Wanker (NY, 1856) T / F
12. Tess Tickle (AR, 1893) T / F
13. Cherry Tart (MS, 1859) T / F
14. Sue Yoo (NY, 2010) T / F
15. Alma Knack (AL, 1982) T / F

Hi (BLANK), I'm Dad

Dad jokes are like regular jokes, only better. The only thing better than a dad joke is a granddad joke. The only thing better than a granddad joke is a great-granddad joke. Fill in the blanks and see what we mean.

1. Your socks are gifts from God because they are so _____.

2. Did you know the _____ got promoted because he was out standing in his field?

3. I had a dream last night that I was a muffler. I woke up _____.

4. That's a very popular _____ because everyone's dying to get in.

5. I left my garbage pail in the sun, and now it's a garbage _____.

6. I don't have a drinking problem. I hardly ever _____.

7. I got fired from my job as a carpenter because I couldn't stop biting my _____.

8. I bought a brown cow because I like _____ milk.

9. You want _____ eggs? Okay. GSEG.

10. My cell died. We are giving it a _____.

11. Did you hear the frog's car broke down? He had to have it _____.

CONTINUED >

12. If your tooth falls out, you can just use _____.

13. I put a cow in the washing machine so we can have a _____.

14. What do you call a deer with no eyes? No _____.

15. When I was a kid, I won a spelling bee. It was impressive but it

_____ me.

exhausted	scarecrow	tan
milkshake	spill	idea
foneral	stung	chocolate
toothpaste	cemetery	scrambled
toad	holy	nails

Bigger Than a Breadbox

Your baby is growing by the week and, for some reason, people like to equate the baby's size to various items you find at a market. It's true. Go week-to-week and unscramble the words to learn how big your grocery bag of joy is getting. When finished, you can also use this as a shopping list.

Week 14: hacep __ __ __ __ __

Week 15: nemol __ __ __ __ __

Week 16: brurbe kucd __ __ __ __ __ __ __ __ __ __

Week 17: nebiae yabb __ __ __ __ __ __ __ __ __ __

Week 18: dosa nac __ __ __ __ __ __ __

Week 19: peiftrgaur __ __ __ __ __ __ __ __ __ __

Week 20: cunocot __ __ __ __ __ __ __

Week 21: neaptuocal __ __ __ __ __ __ __ __ __ __

Week 22: neo dupon feceof gab

__ __ __ __ __ __ __ __ __ __ __ __ __ __ __ __ __ __

Week 23: darbe fola __ __ __ __ __ __ __ __ __

Week 24: dlah nallgo kilm

__ __ __ __ __ __ __ __ __ __ __ __ __ __

Week 25: vefi psnoud lofur

__ __ __ __ __ __ __ __ __ __ __ __ __ __ __

Week 26: dosa trile __ __ __ __ __ __ __ __ __

Week 27: coks komney __ __ __ __ __ __ __ __ __ __

Empathy Exercises

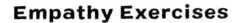

Up until now, most of the complaints a pregnant woman has involve worry, morning sickness, or random aversions. Once the second trimester hits, it's a whole new ballgame.

This is the point when the body transformation starts to kick in. It's like those little figurines you used to buy at the corner store, place in water, and watch grow three times their size overnight. Remember those? If they could talk, they'd tell you they were pretty uncomfortable the whole time.

Admit it. You could never go through it. So, keep your mouth shut as she complains. Nothing you have to offer will ever compare. Express compassion and admiration for the way she is handling her struggle, even if it seems like she's not dealing with it well. No matter how bad her complaints seem to be, they could be (and in many cases should be) much worse.

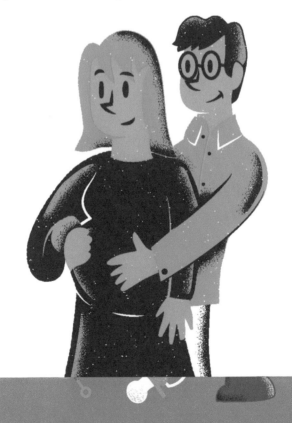

It Does a Body Good

You may live on a steady diet of high-caffeine soda and beef jerky, but a pregnant woman has certain foods that can help her grow the life inside her. Match the foods up to their benefits.

1. Whole grains
2. Salmon
3. Ice cream
4. Spinach
5. Eggs
6. Low-fat yogurt
7. Smurfberries
8. Sweet potatoes
9. The red pill
10. Lean meat
11. Tacos
12. Avocados
13. Scooby Snacks
14. Water
15. Trix cereal

_____ Beta-keratin

_____ Omega-3 fatty acids

_____ Rabbit harassment

_____ Giant forearms, ability to punch bullies across room

_____ Gas

_____ Brain freeze

_____ Hydration

_____ Folic acid and iron

_____ Calcium

_____ Detective abilities

_____ Turn blue; turn mushroom house invisible

_____ Protein

_____ Amino acids

_____ Monosaturated fatty acids

_____ Reveals the Matrix

Papa's Got a Brand-New Bag

Everyone talks about a woman's hospital bag, but what about the dad? Chances are, you're going to be there a while. What should you have ready to go when the big moment arrives?

☐ Phone charger

☐ Phone

☐ Change (or debit card) for the candy/soda machine

☐ Candy and soda, in case there is no machine

☐ Napkins for when you inevitably spill candy and soda all over yourself

☐ A cloth to put over your face in case things get a little, uh, smelly

☐ A book or magazine in case you get no service on your phone

☐ Information needed for insurance/hospital check-in

☐ Headphones

☐ Clean, matching socks

☐ Backup hair stuff (for her) in case she forgets. No one wants to take their picture with bad hair.

☐ A reminder to pick up the flowers and balloons that you are going to order. Trust me.

☐ Whatever food or drink she has been craving for nine months and couldn't have because she was pregnant

Father of Flatulence:
BENJAMIN FRANKLIN

You didn't expect this one, did you? The man most closely credited as the father of farting is the same man credited as the father of electricity. He's the same man on the hundred-dollar bill. How crazy is that?

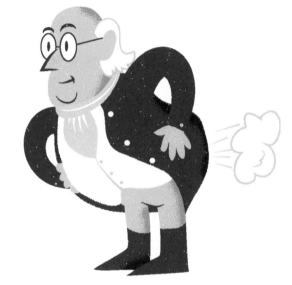

Although people were letting them rip long before he was around, it was Founding Father Ben Franklin who wrote lovingly about the topic in a paper addressed "To the Royal Academy of Farting" in Brussels, Belgium, entitled "Fart Proudly" (seriously). In it, he wrote:

"It is universally well known, that in digesting our common food, there is created or produced in the bowels of human creatures, a great quantity of wind . . . That the permitting of this air to escape and mix with the atmosphere, is usually offensive to the company, from the fetid smell that accompanies it."

Wow. Franklin's reasoning for such a unique topic? To study butt toots for their medical benefits. It wasn't until centuries later that someone else would come along and write a sequel about beans being the magical fruit.

Anazítisi: From the Greek for "Search"

Got a baby name you love? Great! Does it originally mean "butt for face"? If so, you might want to do more research. Read the following clues and then find their matching names in the search box.

Germanic: Will Helmet
Germanic: Whole, Universal
French: Feminine version of Charles
Italian: Mine
Germanic: To Make
Hebrew: Who Is Like God?
Hebrew: Favor, Grace
Dutch: Broken Land
Irish: Little King
Hebrew: Pleasantness
Middle English: Barrel Maker

Latin: Alive
Latin: Clear, Bright, Famous
Greek: Healer
Old English: Pale
Old French: Beloved
Germanic: Ruler of the Army
Hebrew: Friend
Scottish: Little Hollow
Welsh: Great Tide
Old English: Dragon

```
P  U  G  U  Q  D  B  F  S  F  C  P  E  B  S
N  D  S  P  X  R  U  T  H  A  M  M  E  N  O
A  B  R  O  O  K  L  Y  N  H  L  C  U  Y  R
G  A  L  E  K  A  L  B  J  C  E  O  I  V  Y
O  D  Y  L  A  N  K  A  O  G  M  I  N  A  A
L  Q  H  C  V  G  F  O  G  A  Y  S  O  L  N
L  G  Y  C  J  I  P  S  S  Z  R  Z  S  V  B
E  W  T  R  H  E  V  O  P  B  V  W  A  T  H
A  I  F  Z  R  A  N  I  N  N  O  W  J  D  A
H  L  C  A  D  T  R  O  A  N  W  A  D  R  N
C  L  B  C  Q  I  F  L  K  N  I  L  A  A  N
I  I  V  S  G  T  M  U  O  H  M  T  R  K  A
M  A  Z  Z  P  X  A  O  K  T  O  E  A  E  H
T  M  Q  U  F  S  B  I  A  B  T  R  L  M  I
H  E  P  J  Z  Y  D  N  M  N  J  E  C  E  Y
```

On Vacation, Should I Bring . . . ?

Now that you are a dad, you will have the opportunity to express your individual dad style in a number of ways, and create embarrassment for those around you. How will you choose to do so? Consider some of the following:

- Sandals with matching socks?

- Fanny packs with the name of the last city you vacationed in?

- Sun visors that are so tight that they leave a ring around your forehead?

- Sunglasses that rest comfortably on your collar?

- Tokens from Chuck E. Cheese so that you can routinely pull them out at restaurants and ask the kids, *"Do you think they'll take these here?"*

What are some other classic dad accessories you're going to need in your life?

_____

_____

_____

_____

_____

_____

Farewell, Wall Reef

Life before kids will seem like a mixed-up blur. You will need help making sense of it in your head. Study the following paragraph and make sense of the anagrams. Maybe then, you can make sense of who you cone were.

There was a time when you would grab _____ about your

past accomplishments. Those elbow _____ you used to dusty

_____ what made you great. But those days are gone now. Now

the funeral _____ begins, which, as you can see, is a great thing.

Don't silent _____ to the naysayers. Instead, keep your inch

_____ up. You can do any night _____. Life is not a care

_____. It's a serpent _____ from above. It's not something

you ask Satan _____ for at Christmas. It's something you work for

and get your just stressed _____.

Stay Away from My Baby Mama!

There are certain things that are not recommended for a pregnant woman. Review this list and see if you can spot which ones are a danger to your precious cargo.

A Pregnant Woman Should Avoid:

1. **Strenuous exercise** T / F

2. **Candy corn** T / F

3. **Alcohol** T / F

4. **Nickelback** T / F

5. **Smoking** T / F

6. **Raw fish** T / F

7. **Nacho cheese Combos** T / F

8. **Smoked seafood** T / F

9. **Candied yams** T / F

10. **Raw sprouts** T / F

11. **Clam chowder—white, not red** T / F

12. **Powdered donuts** T / F

13. **Cat litter** T / F

14. **Acts of kindness from her partner—hint, dude. Hint.** T / F

15. **Unpasteurized milk or other dairy products** T / F

16. **Hot dogs** T / F

17. **Bubble Yum bubble gum** T / F

Author's Advice

The main thing that they drill in to your head before you leave the hospital is not to shake your baby.

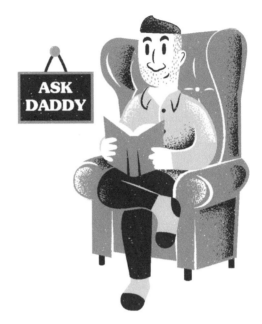

It sounds morbid because we always associate that thought with a purposeful shake. Someone says, *"Don't shake the baby,"* and you get defensive, imagining some nut-ball flinging around infants for fun. In reality, though, they are right to caution you because, well, rocking a baby is pretty darn close to shaking them.

There's a reason there's a rock-a-bye song for newborns. It's because they like it. An infant, struggling to sleep, will gently fall into slumber as you glide them back and forth in your arms. If your arms are full, they sell mechanical swings that do the same trick. They're worth every penny.

A crying baby might settle down when you rock them faster, and that's where the danger lies. There's a thin line between "rock" and "shake." Don't overdo a manic bedtime routine. Keep everything smooth, and imagine yourself in the baby's position, being swung in the arms of a giant monster 15 times your size. Like all things in life, just don't overdo it.

Scrambled Life Lessons

You want to do what's right by your kid. We all do. Life lessons, though, can sometimes be confusing. Read the advice and unscramble the effect it will have on your kid. Get it wrong, and your kid might end up toony lunes.

1. Help those less fortunate—aherbticla __ __ __ __ __ __ __ __ __ __

2. Treat others as you would want to be treated—ekindssn

   __ __ __ __ __ __ __ __

3. Stand up for yourself—gerucao __ __ __ __ __ __ __

4. Study hard—ceietnlleing __ __ __ __ __ __ __ __ __ __

5. Play fair—ohspsrsmitpna __ __ __ __ __ __ __ __ __ __ __

6. Care about others' feelings—spaosncimo

   __ __ __ __ __ __ __ __ __

7. Play hard, work hard—thenstrg __ __ __ __ __ __ __ __

8. Take a joke—rumho __ __ __ __ __

9. Keep a clean workspace—raiotznganio

   __ __ __ __ __ __ __ __ __ __ __

10. Work up a sweat regularly and eat right—infests

    __ __ __ __ __ __

11. Stand by your friends—yaotlyl __ __ __ __ __ __ __

12. Keep a secret—tuhtoswrsrnteis

    __ __ __ __ __ __ __ __ __ __ __ __ __ __

13. Stand by your word—tauflhif __ __ __ __ __ __ __ __

14. Accept your faults—myhltiui __ __ __ __ __ __ __ __

15. Love your dad—opcteerfni __ __ __ __ __ __ __ __ __ __

Father of The Jock Strap:
C. F. BENNETT

It was a bumpy road for bikers before C. F. Bennett put a strap around their waists and a cup around their junk. Working for a Chicago sporting goods company, Sharp & Smith, Bennett was able to give men across the world peace of mind with his invention, aimed to protect their most delicate of areas from the rigors of sports mishaps. Without him, there would be far fewer babies in the world and far more sopranos singing choir music.

Originally called the "Bike Jockey Strap," Bennett's gift to the privates was first introduced in 1874. Eventually, Bennett's brand became a company unto itself, and "Bike" owned everything strap until they were purchased in 2003 by Russell Athletics. You could say that Russell was on their jocks from that day on.

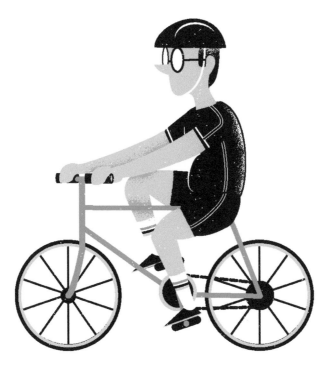

Get Your Dad On

Superman has a cape. Mr. Rogers has a sweater. Batman has a belt thing. If you're going to be a dad, you need to make sure you have your dad-pack packed, if you know what I mean. Carry this list with you and check off the items as you put them in your Dad Cave. You have a Dad Cave, right? Ugh. Okay. Add it to the list!

- ☐ Dad Cave (A private spot to hide out.)
- ☐ Screwdrivers (Phillips. Most toys now have Phillips-head screws blocking the batteries.)
- ☐ Single dollar bills, coins
- ☐ Gum/candy
- ☐ A calculator (It makes you seem old and wise . . . an abacus also works.)
- ☐ Coffee . . . tons of coffee
- ☐ Spare car keys
- ☐ Spare remote control
- ☐ Tylenol
- ☐ Sunglasses (One pair for style, one pair for blocking sun—you will only use the latter as time moves on.)

- ☐ Knee-high black socks
- ☐ Cargo shorts, many
- ☐ A shirt that says "DAD" somewhere on it
- ☐ A funny wig that you pair with a high-pitched voice to ask your kid, *"Where is your dad? Have you seen him?"* Ha! They love it!
- ☐ Swiss Army knife
- ☐ Batteries . . . tons of batteries: AA, AAA, C, D, Lithium
- ☐ Tape measure
- ☐ Crown (You will wear it, often ironically, more than you realize.)

Searching for a New Life

Use the clues to find words associated with things that will, at the very least, be curtailed once you add "Daddy" to your résumé.

Used to be eight hours, now it's three.

Short spurts, mostly in the bathroom.

Ten more bags, no longer a whim.

Costs an extra $50 for a high school kid to eat your food.

You don't go to these anymore; you enjoy them in 15-minute clips at home before passing out.

Shhhh, this disappears for years.

This used to rarely be on your clothes, now they're part of every outfit.

Up and down, up and down, all this lifting causes havoc on this.

There was once a time when these things were thrown at you for fun.

At one time, you may have hit this. Now you sterilize and give this.

You once had tons of this loose in your pockets, now it's something you have to do every few hours.

This is your new alarm clock.

You never had to check your shoulder for this before you started holding a baby over it.

```
H  J  R  I  V  R  T  E  E  R  P  O  J  D  L
R  E  U  U  O  K  G  B  A  T  T  K  E  F  M
W  A  U  R  L  R  G  F  P  E  H  K  R  G  F
A  L  V  C  O  D  A  R  I  G  P  F  M  M  A
T  E  Z  G  C  D  I  U  J  Q  X  O  M  V  P
V  C  K  P  S  V  Q  G  X  W  V  X  I  G  J
E  A  W  U  A  T  N  I  U  I  B  N  V  W  S
Q  B  C  C  P  I  L  P  E  D  Z  Z  O  J  Y
N  O  Y  A  Y  Q  C  S  E  E  D  B  O  C  O
Y  T  G  R  T  K  S  Z  X  E  G  R  R  B  T
B  T  C  V  B  I  W  T  P  H  L  N  L  Q  S
A  L  P  A  J  U  O  L  A  Q  F  S  A  V  U
C  E  Q  X  W  K  D  N  L  I  Z  N  A  H  D
K  A  P  Y  N  P  J  M  C  Q  N  F  H  P  C
X  U  U  D  A  T  E  S  O  R  U  S  W  I  H
```

Author's Advice

You're halfway through the pregnancy at this point and, well, there is going to be some stress. That's normal.

Unfortunately, you have to hold yourself together around the mom-to-be because stressing her is the exact opposite of what you want to have happen. That is actually what you'll find yourself mostly stressed about. Just like it's hard to get experience without getting a job and hard to get a job without experience, this is one of life's great paradoxes. You are stressed about worrying your baby's mother, but expressing it causes the very worry that you're stressed about. Argh!

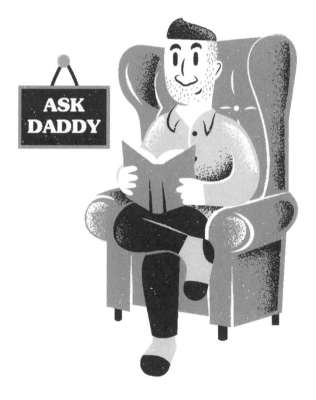

(BLANK) This

You can't give good advice if you don't know good advice. Here is a list of solid words of wisdom every poppa should know. Fill in the missing words. Because nothing in life is handed to you! Hey, that's another one!

1. _____ me once, shame on you. _____ me twice, shame on me.

2. Don't _____ on an electric fence.

3. Only _____ people say they're bored.

4. Two wrongs don't make a right, but three _____ do.

5. Ask a man with one _____ for directions. He knows the easiest route.

6. There's plenty of _____ in the sea, but you have to get past the litter.

7. Happy wife, happy _____.

8. Put something in your _____, not on it.

9. When life hands you lemons, _____ them.

10. There's no "I" in _____.

11. Neither a _____ nor a _____ be.

12. Be _____ today than you were yesterday.

13. There's no such thing as _____ shrimp.

free	fool	fish
pee	better	team
life	lender	sell
lefts	fool	boring
head	leg	borrower

A Tale as Old as Dad

We all want to be great dads. The following story is one that guides you through that journey. Do your best to unscramble some of the words and phrases to correct the meaning and to give it a happy ending.

A admirer _____ man may be nervous becoming a dad. He knows

it will affect everyone's elvis _____. Sure, everyone might say, "nail

biting refreshes the feet" _____ but in

reality, the mage of file _____ _____ _____ costs

you a lot of hard work. It's important to silent _____ and come out

of it being able to say, yes—I learned words _____ _____

_____—that is me. Whether you have a little princess or an old guy

_____ _____, you will show your child that home, from the

boredom _____ to the thicken _____, doesn't have to be

seen as a hacks _____ . No matter the size, it can be your cleats

_____. Make sure your skid _____ know that when you

close that odor _____, they are loved and raced _____

for. One day, you will turn around and find that baby is now a generate

_____, their thermos _____ will be nether guy ivory

_____ _____ and you, well, you'll be more than the head

of the should hoe _____. You'll be a lap _____, a meat

_____, and maybe even a finder _____ to the end.

The Poop Scoop

This isn't a maybe. Your house is *definitely* going to smell. You have a little person pooping constantly in your home now. What do you do with the diaper after a changing? Do you burn it and sacrifice it to the Gods of Doo-Doo? No. You put it in a bucket thing and leave it in your house for too long. How long is too long? Any length of time is too long.

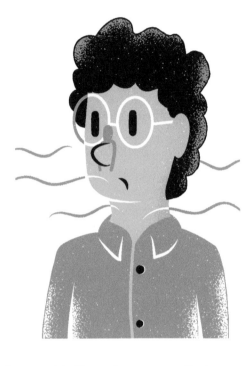

There's nothing you can do to prevent it. Potty training doesn't happen for years. The best you can do is get ahead of it all. Sprays, air fresheners, and those garbage bags with lilac pictures on their boxes help. There are many precautions you can take and, if you are serious about not being a stinker, you should take them.

The most important thing is to know that this is inevitable. It doesn't take long to go "nose blind" to the odor of baby lingering in the air. You might not smell it, but the rest of the world does. If you're cool with that, then embrace it. Also, maybe buy some stock in air fresheners.

Delivering Your (NOUN)

You may think your wife's OBGYN has a strange personality. They are, after all, people. People can be weird. If you buy into this line of thinking, fill out the following *Storytime!* and read it out loud. After you do, you'll feel better about the OBGYN you have.

1. Halloween candy_____

2. Strong verb ending in -ing_____

3. Room in the house_____

4. Electronic devices_____

5. Verb_____

6. Piece of clothing_____

7. Infamous celebrity_____

8. Animal_____

9. Crazy nickname_____

10. Verb_____

11. Body part_____

12. Something made of metal_____

13. Farm animal_____

14. Breakfast items_____

15. Nouns_____

16. Adjective_____

CONTINUED >

Hello! This is a welcome email to the mommy and daddy to be. My name is Dr. 1._____, and I will be 2._____ a baby out of y'all! Yee-haw!

First, some rules. I would like you to arrive at my 3._____ at least 40 minutes before your appointment. For your pleasure, I have installed 4._____ around the waiting area. Do not touch them, 5._____ them, or put them in your mouth. If you must, I ask that you wear a 6._____ on your hands. These devices are expensive. They once belonged to 7._____.

I also ask that you do not tell anyone about the 8._____ that is sitting in the front of the building. His name is 9._____, and he tells me what to do. If he suspects that we have been discussing him, he might 10._____ me in the 11._____ with a rusty 12._____.

Good luck! I can't wait to yank that little 13._____ from y'all. My fee for this is $40 and ten 14._____ wrapped with a bow.

Love and 15._____,

Your 16._____ Doctor

Paging Doctor Google: Breech

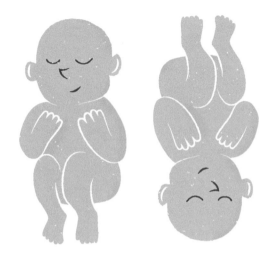

If you play video games, you've heard the term "breach." Shouting it out loud brings up visions of *Call of Duty* soldiers screaming at you as the enemy team runs into your headquarters. You panic. You shoot a claymore on the ground, blowing up your teammates. It causes you to rage quit by kicking the controller across the room. When you log back in, you get a voice message from a ten-year-old that is meaner than anything any adult has ever said to you. Yikes.

In terms of pregnancy, a "breech" (note the spelling difference) means that the baby is positioned with their butt down where their head ought to be in the womb at the time of delivery. It sounds scary, and, while not optimal, it's not nearly as awful as it seems. The only similarity to video games is the panic it stirs inside when an OBGYN says it to you during a routine appointment.

There are ways to deliver a baby in breech, so everything will usually work out fine. But be prepared to hear it. This is the time when people start to randomly mention it in passing as a possibility, sometimes when relatives tell you their own birthing stories. Just don't shoot any claymores and you should be fine.

Dirty Diaper, Filled Butt Pillow

A lot of parenting is, uh, pretty gross. Phrases need to be softened so relatives don't vomit when you say them out loud. Because then someone else will throw up and then you have to clean that up too, and that's gross. It's a whole thing. Match the gross activity to its sweeter phrasing.

1. Baby Vomit
2. Wet Baby
3. Filled Diaper
4. Snot
5. Eye Mucus
6. Gas
7. Spit-Up
8. Soiled Diapers
9. Wet Sheets
10. Crusty Pacifiers
11. Dirty Diaper
12. Umbilical Stump
13. Drool
14. Slimy Hands
15. Bathtub Poop

_____ Wee-Wee Pads

_____ Nummies Sequel

_____ S.S. *Floatie Doo-Doo*

_____ Boogz

_____ Little Mister (or Miss) Stinker Pants

_____ Lil' Soggy Bottom

_____ Teeny Slippery Fingers

_____ Baby Unplugged

_____ Leaky Lil' Face

_____ Squooshy Tooshie

_____ Peeper Creepers

_____ Stinky Binkies

_____ Spittle

_____ Little Presents

_____ Premium Unleaded Baby Fuel

What Can I Do to Raise My Kid to Be . . . ?

As a dad, you will have so much influence on your child. Taking that into consideration, what can you do to raise your kid to be the:

Leader of the country?

_____

Leader of the school?

_____

Leader of a street gang called the "Monkey Ghouls"?

_____

Leader of a secret society that controls the world from its shadowy headquarters?

_____

A WWE Intercontinental Champion?

_____

Leader of a family as strong and wonderful as ours?

_____

_____

What the Frig!

If not for bad words, some people would say no words at all. When you have a child, for some reason, those words are the ones most easily duplicated. For that reason, it's important to know what the bad words are—no matter the language. Read the words below and mark whether each one is a true curse word or not. Go on. Don't be a dinglebeard.

1. **Himmeldonnerwetter** T / F

2. **Tantolone** T / F

3. **Merde** T / F

4. **Smergalop** T / F

5. **Silbabot** T / F

6. **Tring-Pol** T / F

7. **Skitstovel** T / F

8. **Buckobat** T / F

9. **Teezak hamra** T / F

10. **Wilosperay** T / F

11. **Branleur** T / F

12. **Gobblygooker** T / F

13. **Kisama** T / F

14. **Porkenbeen** T / F

In This Trimester

Yeah, this is the time when a baby bump becomes a baby bada-bumpa-bump. Not only does the woman's stomach grow, but so do her hands and ankles. Some women even have changes to their facial structure (especially the nose). It happens. Don't get crazy about it. After all, you had a hand (or more) in doing it.

The important thing to know is that the mommy-to-be is going to be self-conscious. Try to remember that. Between the cramps, aches, body changes, and hormones, she has a long list of reasons to feel not-her-best. You do not. In fact, if you want to be a good partner, this is an easy place to step up.

Be nice. Be complimentary. Don't point out changes that are more obvious to her than to anyone else. She is doing something incredibly hard that you literally cannot do, but will benefit from for the rest of your life. Show you appreciate it. Things will go back to normal in nine months, and when they do, you'll have a family to show for it.

Stuck In One Spot

When you think of rocking your baby to sleep, you imagine a serene setting of parental bliss. What no one tells you is that usually the slightest move turns peace into chaos. So, you might find yourself stuck, with your arms folded, for quite some time. Best prepare now. You're going to need:

☐ A comfortable chair (preferably a rocker)

☐ A pillow for your butt (if the rocker is a wooden one)

☐ A blanket (for you, not the baby)

☐ A neck pillow in case you fall asleep (Who am I kidding? For when you *definitely* fall asleep)

☐ A phone charger; it might be a while

☐ A hands-free system of turning on and off lights (Alexa, Google, fairy, genie)

☐ A sleeping area for the baby in close proximity

☐ A non-squeaky floor (trust us on this one)

☐ If you are the owner of a squeaky floor, mental notes on where the squeaks are so you can two-step around them

☐ A baby monitor near the area (both for watching the baby and for calling for help)

☐ A window to look out of like a puppy on a rainy day

Author's Advice

It's been said before,
but it is worth repeating:
you are probably feeling
overwhelmed. Trust me
on this one, there will be
people weighing in to
offer advice.

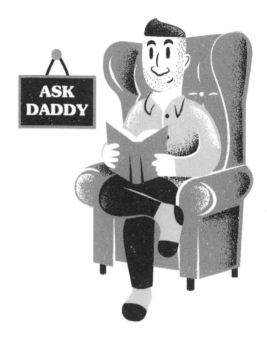

People will be giving
you plenty of advice,
and, by all means, take
it. Listen to what they
tell you and keep mental
notes on all the tips you
pick up along the way.
The things your grand-
parents did for your
parents, while dated
in their delivery (who has an icebox these days?), still hold up in
execution.

All that being true, remember one thing above all else. Trust
your gut. You're the dad now. If you feel like there's a way to do
something, do it. When you have a child, your paternal instincts
kick in, and those instincts are very real. They may be new. They
may be based on intuition. They all, though, are real. This is your
kid. As long as you feel you're doing what is best for them, that's
what you should do.

Sometimes you can map out your reasoning and present it to
others in a clearly defined and easy to understand way. But if not,
sometimes the reason is a simple one that most fathers are used
to saying: *'Cause I'm the Daddy. That's why.*

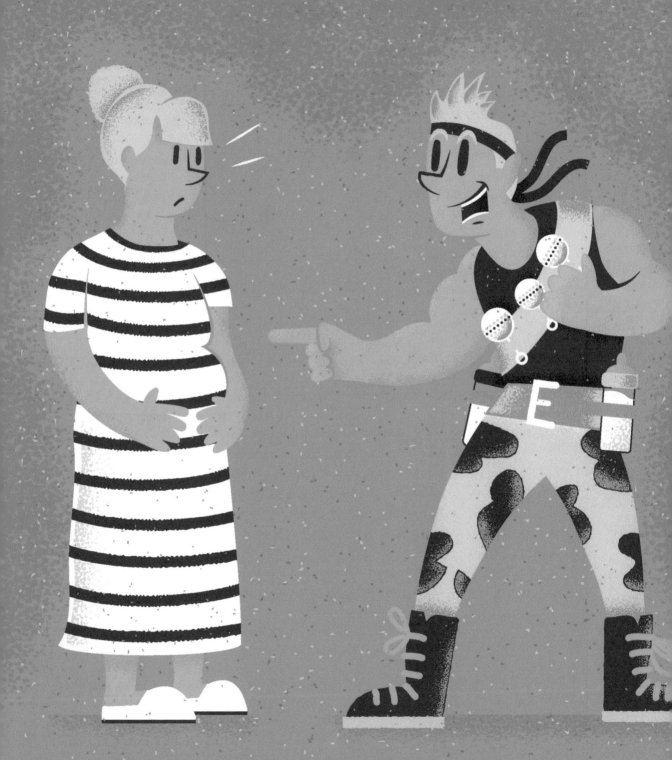

PART THREE

Last Trimester (Weeks 28–40)

This is it. You made it. It's the fourth quarter. It's the bottom of the ninth. It's the twelfth round. It's the third trimester.

By now, you will be significantly fatigued from pregnancy and want nothing more than to be holding a baby in your arms. You can see those days clearer now than you could in the opening weeks. You've been asked so often if you're ready that you now feel like you are. That's good. You should, and even if you don't, you *are* ready. You'll see. Fatherhood is just around the corner, and once pregnancy is over, there will be a whole laundry list of new insanities to learn about. But that is then. This is now.

Now is the time for many of the stereotypes you've heard about when it comes to pregnant partners and baby prep to manifest themselves before your eyes. It's time to really buckle down, strap in, and prepare for the launch of your next generation. Time's a-tickin', and the water's about to be a breakin'. Put on your swim shoes; it's time for the final part of the pregnancy trilogy. Prepare for *Trimester III: Electric Baby Boogaloo*.

Grand, Father

Have you started thinking about grandparent names? You should. This can be a major decision for many families. Grandmoms and pops can get pretty demanding. Make sure you know your choices. There is a fine line between cutesy names for parental parents and insults from a Steven Seagal movie. Don't believe it? See if you can figure out which of these are synonyms for grandparents and which ones are street-tough insults. Good luck, Gumba.

1. **Nono** ____

2. **Momo** ____

3. **Poppy** ____

4. **Paunchy** ____

5. **Grammy** ____

6. **Fanoke** ____

7. **Pappy** ____

8. **Crappy** ____

9. **Nana** ____

10. **Chump Stain** ____

11. **Mimi** ____

12. **Mook** ____

13. **Yaya** ____

14. **Yo-yo** ____

15. **Baba** ____

16. **Palooka** ____

17. **Gigi** ____

18. **Jadrool** ____

19. **Ommy** ____

20. **Jabrone** ____

Third Try, Mister

Okay. Two quizzes down and one last one to go. You should know how quizzes work by now. Get these wrong and, well, you should feel ashamed.

1. **What is a C-section?**
   a) The area under the bridge
   b) Part of the arena with the third-to-best view of the stage
   c) $738 plus cost of the motel room
   d) A surgical procedure used to deliver a baby through incisions in the abdomen and uterus

2. **Forceps are:**
   a) The part that they cut at a bris
   b) One more than three ceps
   c) Two for a dollar at the grocery store
   d) A handheld, hinged instrument used during some deliveries for grasping and holding objects

3. **The third trimester begins:**
   a) At 28 weeks
   b) After spring break
   c) When someone screams "*TOGA!*"
   d) On the count of three. One . . . two . . .

4. **A baby's bones really begin to grow in the third trimester. So, it is important for the mom to eat lots of:**
   a) Calcium
   b) Baby bones
   c) Dog bones
   d) Pac Man cereal

5. **By this trimester, the baby's skin becomes:**
   a) Opaque
   b) Purple
   c) Delicious
   d) Scaly, like a dinosaur tail

6. **In the third trimester, your baby develops all five:**
   a) Senses
   b) Little ducks
   c) Jackson brothers
   d) Ears (three fall off prior to birth)

CONTINUED >

7. **The temporary organ that connects a developing fetus via the umbilical cord to the uterine wall is called:**
    a) Uh, what? Oh my God.
    b) Charlie Tuna
    c) The baby tape
    d) Placenta

8. **It is not uncommon for a woman's breasts during this trimester to become:**
    a) Leaky
    b) Purple
    c) Upside-down
    d) Scaly, like Charlie Tuna

9. **Some women complain that when sneezing during this trimester, they might accidentally:**
    a) Release the ghost of Zuul
    b) Levitate
    c) Shart
    d) Pee

10. **The sign that you are ready to go to the hospital for delivery is usually when:**
    a) The timer goes off
    b) The baby sends you a text
    c) Your partner's water breaks
    d) You just can't take it anymore

11. **As the baby "drops" inside a mother towards the end of pregnancy, she can appear to be:**
    a) Waddling
    b) A Weeble-Wobble
    c) A bowling pin
    d) Danny Devito

12. **As your baby's brain grows in this trimester, they will start to:**
    a) Do your taxes
    b) Use telekinesis
    c) Blink
    d) Slide into other babies' DMs

Baby Froop

Pregnancy seems as if it lasts forever, but, in hindsight, it zips by. Baby-raising is the same way. Before long, your little bundle of joy will be a wobbling accident waiting to happen. Read the following passage and solve the anagrams to learn how to protect your child by baby proofing. But hurry up!

Babies are underflow _____. We all know that. But they are

also constantly in noseguard _____ situations. It is up to us,

the shafter _____ to keep them safe. For example, downing

belch _____ is a big no-no. You have to lock that up or put it

on a high flesh _____. That way you won't wind up dealing with

dance tics _____. It is also a good idea to lock up anything

harps _____ or else you might wind up seeing your kid get a

cranial toe _____. No one wants that. Finally, be very careful of

enemas flop _____ _____. Between the foreskin dame

_____ _____ _____, you could be looking at

lube rot _____. Always have a sexier figure hit _____

_____ on hand. You'll be glad you did.

Father of the Man Cave: JOHN GRAY

The birth of the term "Man Cave" is usually credited to the 1992 book *Men Are from Mars, Women Are from Venus* by John Gray. In it, Gray suggests that the human male has a need "to withdraw to his cave when overwhelmed by stresses."

It would have been nice if he had called for something a bit more luxurious, as the thought of a cave brings up imagery from desert wars and battle cries, but we'll take it. The Man Cave is a corny term for a much-needed retreat from the everyday. Without it, more dads would go the way of Jack Torrance in *The Shining* instead of Mr. Rogers. And, as we all know, all work and no cave makes Jack a dull boy.

Due to the popularity of his book, Gray eventually opened the Mars Venus Institute and Counseling Centers, forcing men to come out of their caves and to share their feelings. Many men obliged because, without him, we'd all be stuck in the family room with people bugging us. Thank you, John Gray. Our neon beer signs, signed sports jerseys, and electronic dart boards hidden in a back office of the house thank you, too!

A Rose by Any Other Name

What's in a name? Letters. (That's a Dad Joke—get used to 'em, Pops.) For many celebrities, there was a great deal of success in establishing new monikers as fame found them. Now, you find them. Match the originals to their well-known identities. It only takes a few vowel movements (that's another Dad Joke).

1. Bruno Mars
2. Jamie Foxx
3. Rihanna
4. Lady Gaga
5. Nicki Minaj
6. Frank Ocean
7. Drake
8. Ludacris
9. Gerald Ford
10. Vin Diesel
11. Charlie Sheen
12. Meg Ryan
13. David Bowie
14. Marilyn Manson
15. Floyd Mayweather
16. Seal
17. Method Man
18. The Ultimate Warrior
19. Carrot Top
20. Kareem Abdul-Jabbar

_____ Mark Sinclair

_____ Peter Hernandez

_____ Ferdinand Lewis Alcindor Jr.

_____ Eric Bishop

_____ Carlos Estevez

_____ Scott Thompson

_____ Robyn Fenty

_____ Jim Hellwig

_____ Stefani Germanotta

_____ Clifford Smith Jr.

_____ Onika Maraj

_____ Christopher Cooksey

_____ Henry Samuel

_____ Aubrey Graham

_____ Floyd Joy Sinclair

_____ Christopher Bridges

_____ Leslie King Jr.

_____ Brian Warner

_____ Margaret Hyra

_____ David Jones

Watch Your Language

Sometimes it's hard to make it through a damn sentence without cursing. But when you become a dad, you need to substitute certain words in order to avoid notes home from school. You'll need to start early. No one picks up a four-letter word quicker than a three-year-old. Find these convenient dad curses that will come in handy when you are just dying to say . . . oh, you know.

SunnyLaBeach   Fudgebrownies   RingoStarr   Fandango
Funcoland   Ballbearings   CopaCabana   FalafelWaffles
Beachballs   Sheetshack   LasikEyeSurgery
Dipstick   Dictaphone   DonkeyCrackers
Weenis   SmothersBrother   Constantinople

```
E F Q V Z V S R E K C A R C Y E K N O D
O A R J G I E V G D C N Q M S S L H V S
P L I O G N A D N A F S U A L U O A M S
C A N E H H U M A H E I A L X L T O Y H
A F G I N L Q Z H I E N A W D C T Y O E
C E O S E S A K S U Y B O Y D H G F V E
F L S M V U H S P G H N V H E Q C T H T
U W T D S L O S I C N S F R P O K C V S
D A A N Y P W F A K W I S X N A A S F H
G F R A Q T F E J L E B R S U E T D M A
E F R L D Q B C V S R Y T A B P I C X C
B L E O D R O V O O Y A E A E P I Z I K
R E U C C T Y Q T P N B L S S B E F X D
O S Y N W H O H O T A Y X T U C L Y G I
W L T U W C E T I Q N C I I S R M L D N
N D J F A R B N Q N J C A S L Y G Y A L
I I F L V S O O U D K X H B H S D E W B
E X L R Y P I S M O X Y G F A H Y V R M
S M Z O L S I N E E W B T M P N Y I J Y
J T S E E W J Q F I R J X V V I A O Z Q
```

Author's Advice

You are going to be tempted to take short-cuts on baby proofing. After all, you ate paint as a kid, and you're fine, right? Headaches, sleep-walking, and cannibalism notwithstanding.

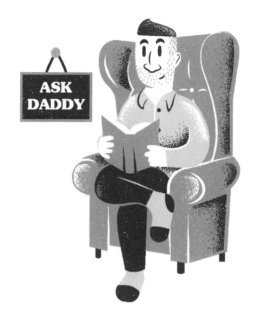

A piece of advice—don't cut corners on this. If you do, your baby will cut themselves on those jagged corners. If there is any way for a baby to get hurt, that baby will find it. When they do, everyone will look at you with a dissatisfied glare and ask you point blank:

"Weren't you watching them?"

Yes. You were. You watched your kid run, headfirst, into the corner of the table. You even watched as they fell back in tears. It took your paint-addled brain a minute to process the scene.

Just as pregnancy ended before you knew it, that little bundle of baby will be mobile before you know it. The sooner you get ahead of life's little pitfalls, the sooner you can ensure that your kid will be in one piece by the time school starts.

Remember, no shelf is high enough and no possible danger is low-key enough to keep tiny fingers from reaching. If you don't keep an eye out for those tiny fingers, there will end up being fewer fingers than when you started.

Happily Never After

Kids like movies. Those movies are kind of nuts. How nuts? You don't even know. Oh, you do? Prove it. Match the "family film" to its insane plot.

1. *The Wizard of Oz*
2. *Toy Story*
3. *Snow White*
4. *Frozen*
5. *Sesame Street*
6. *The NeverEnding Story*
7. *Mary Poppins*
8. *Beauty and the Beast*
9. *The Little Mermaid*
10. *Pinocchio*
11. *It's a Wonderful Life*
12. *Charlie and the Chocolate Factory*

_____ Monster forces girl to live with him. Love story.

_____ Flying nanny encourages children to self-medicate with sugar.

_____ Kid watches other children die on factory tour. Enjoys songs from indentured servants.

_____ Girl kills longtime resident. Sets out with three friends to kill her sister.

_____ Two sisters. One has a problem with ice.

_____ Girl gets poisoned. A group of miners keep her in the woods. A stranger kisses her without her consent.

_____ Man gives up on his dreams. Tries to kill himself on Christmas. Fails.

_____ Old man pretends wooden doll is his son.

_____ Inanimate objects fight. Nearly get killed by neighbor. Battle for the love of a little boy.

_____ Residents of inner city struggle with addiction and literacy. One neighbor lives in a trash can.

_____ Octopus takes girl's voice. Forces her to trick sailor into marriage.

_____ Boy gets bullied. Reads book. Rides giant dog. Watches horse drown in mud.

DIY Storytime

You need to know bedtime stories. Chances are, you don't. No worries, Grimm, you can make up your own. Go on. Give it a try. You'll live happily ever after.

1. Adjective_____

2. Type of plant_____

3. Location_____

4. Verb_____

5. Type of sandwich bread_____

6. Lunch meat_____

7. Body part_____

8. Dessert_____

9. Verb_____

10. Verb (past tense)_____

11. Body part_____

12. Fruit_____

13. Sharp object (plural)_____

14. Favorite album_____

CONTINUED >

DIY Storytime CONTINUED

Once upon a time, there lived a 1._____ princess named Princess

2._____. She was the most beautiful girl in all the 3._____. Her favorite

thing to do was to 4._____ with all the little elves in the neighboring village.

Then, one day, the evil Lord 5._____ arrived with his evil 6._____

of doom and aimed it right at the princess. She screamed and clutched her

7._____, but alas, it was too late. He had turned her into a 8._____.

Now, she was defenseless as he 9._____ beside her. Luckily, the elves saw

what was happening and 10._____ the evildoer in the 11._____ with

their secret weapon—a seven-foot 12._____ wrapped in 13._____. Once

they were done, they used magic to transform the princess back and save the day.

She was so happy that she gave them all 14._____ as a thank you.

Say This/Not That

They say that it's not what you say, but how you say it. That's true, but it's kinda also what you say. It's both. Use the clues below to figure out what word you should substitute when talking to your (very) pregnant and (very) sensitive partner.

ACROSS

1. Horny
3. Annoying
4. Mean
7. Picky
9. Angry
11. Lazy

DOWN

2. Boring
3. Forceful
5. Cranky
6. Crazy
8. Sweaty
10. Gluttonous

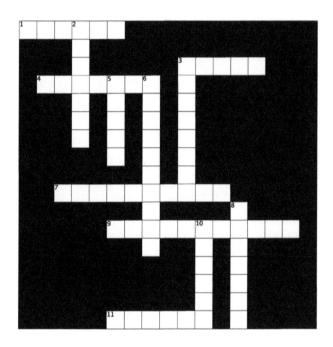

The Poop Scoop

Life is full of questions that aren't really questions. They are questions with hidden agendas.

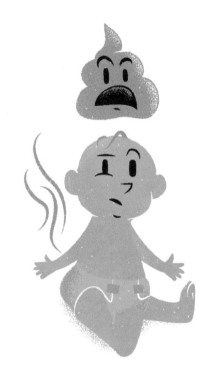

Now that you're going to be a dad, get used to a new one. Ready?

"Do we have any more diapers?"

That is a loaded question unlike any you have ever heard before or ever will again. No person on Earth thinks that a dad is hoarding diapers in his man cave. Your partner knows damn well you don't have any diapers.

She's asking because you need to go out and buy more. Usually, by the time she asks, it's an emergency. There's a baby, covered in baby waste, squirming around on a table with nothing to cover them up. So, you have to make a speed run to the pharmacy. Time's a-wasting.

The lesson here? Be prepared. Have lots of diapers on hand *before* the baby comes home. You're going to need 'em. The last thing you want to hear is that question . . . especially if you're busy chugging your early-morning vodka.

In Your Dreams

Another perk of a woman's third trimester is that she has crazy dreams and gets to tell her partner all about her crazy dreams. So be prepared to hear some nutty stuff. But listening isn't fun without a story or two of your own. Use the *Storytime!* below to make up your own batshit crazy dream to tell her.

1. Obscure job title_____

2. Foreign country_____

3. Friend you don't talk to_____

4. Room in the house_____

5. Color_____

6. Type of fabric_____

7. Song lyric_____

8. Nonsense chant_____

9. Piece of furniture_____

10. Animal_____

11. Body part_____

12. Liquid_____

13. Four-syllable word_____

14. Piece of clothing_____

15. Food_____

CONTINUED >

In Your Dreams CONTINUED

So, I was working as a 1._____ in 2._____ for 3._____.

We were both sitting in a 4._____, but it was all a weird 5._____

and decorated in 6._____. So, I hear this voice that keeps saying

"7._____" and I go, "What?" Then it goes, "8._____." So

now I'm freaked out. I get up, look under the 9._____ and see a

10._____, only it has this giant 11._____. So I squeeze it, and

all this 12._____ comes out. Then we dipped brushes in it and painted

the word "13._____" all over the walls and on our chests. Then my

14._____ turned into 15._____ and we ate it. Then I woke up and

thought about how great you are. You're great. Aw. Thanks for having my baby.

Goodbye Yedboog

Your life is about to change, and many things that you have come to love will soon be nothing but scrambled memories. Unscramble them one last time. Then . . . say "goodbye."

- Lepes   __ __ __ __ __

- Icen Cetholc   __ __ __ __ __ __ __ __ __ __ __

- Ricpyva   __ __ __ __ __ __ __

- Arnpiygt   __ __ __ __ __ __ __ __

- Lacen Hemo   __ __ __ __ __ __ __ __ __ __

- Scilene   __ __ __ __ __ __ __

- Yomen   __ __ __ __ __

- Anudoesgr Soty   __ __ __ __ __ __ __ __ __ __ __ __ __

- Staf Scar   __ __ __ __ __ __ __ __

- Azcyr Serdnif   __ __ __ __ __ __ __ __ __ __ __ __

- Zyal Orgmnisn   __ __ __ __ __ __ __ __ __ __ __ __

- Rab Things   __ __ __ __ __ __ __ __ __

- Kregges   __ __ __ __ __ __ __

- Shwim   __ __ __ __ __

- Stal Etimun Strip

  __ __ __ __ __ __ __ __ __ __ __ __ __ __ __

- Nimgron Exs   __ __ __ __ __ __ __ __ __ __

Paging Doctor Google:
Cord Blood Bank

Shortly after your baby is
born, someone will come
around asking about
"cord blood banking." This
sounds like something out
of a vampire movie, but
it's far more innocent than
it seems.

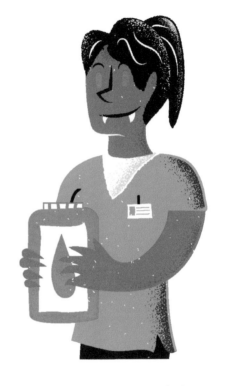

Cord blood banking is
when the hospital takes
the blood from your baby's
clamped umbilical cord,
freezes it, and stores it for
later use. In the event that
your baby gets sick, this
unused blood can come in
handy due to its richness
of cells and other needed
materials. It's that simple.

OK. So, it doesn't sound as simple or innocent as I made it out
to be. It sounds involved, bizarre, and a little . . . gross. I get it. Just
know that this is something people do and something that you
will be asked about when you arrive for delivery. Most dads know
little to nothing about it beforehand. You? You're different. You
read about it here and probably made a wincing face similar to
the one you made when watching *The Human Centipede*. That's
cool. No one is judging your face. It's your baby's scrumptious
umbilical blood they are after.

(There's that face again.)

Before You Name Them . . .

Before settling on a name, there are some things to consider. You and your partner should definitely talk about the following. Is the name:

☐ Shared by an ex?

☐ Shared by the pet of someone you know?

☐ Shared by a serial killer?

☐ Shared by someone you and your friends have mocked relentlessly?

☐ Shared by someone who has mocked you or your friends relentlessly?

☐ Shared by a shamed celebrity?

☐ Shared by a corny celebrity?

☐ Shared by a TV/movie character who your kid might be mocked for?

☐ Easily rhymed with something terribly dirty?

☐ Rhymed with your partner's or your last name?

☐ Combined with your partner's or your last name to make a funny word?

☐ A pun?

☐ A curse word in a foreign language?

A World Full of Bosj

Tom's son was always trying to ham it up. Luckily, he grew up to be a

famous taroc _____. It was natural, though, as he always had

fancied himself an strait _____ himself and had tried his hand as

a creditor _____ early in life. His neighbor, Bill, had a daughter

who went on to stinted _____ school. That's where she met an

outraced _____ who changed her life and inspired her to chase

her real dreams of being moray _____ of a small city. Of course,

she had to wait until after she was done being a stunted _____

and, after years of work as a wariest _____ and even a small stint

as a lewder _____, she achieved her dream. Thank goodness that

cheater _____ was there to guide the way. Otherwise, she might

have turned out to be a patier _____, like her dad. That would

have been wild. After all, she has both eyes and doesn't even own a raptor

_____!

A (ADJECTIVE) Baby Announcement

You've just had a baby. You're tired. Use this form to get the news out. Don't worry. It'll make sense. They'll get it.

1. Vegetable (plural)_____
2. Random date_____
3. Random time_____
4. Random place_____
5. Emotion_____
6. Cartoon character_____
7. Color_____
8. Your partner's last name_____
9. One-word insult_____
10. Toiletry item_____
11. Adjective_____
12. Verb (past tense)_____
13. Creature_____
14. Distant relative_____
15. Barnyard animal_____
16. Movie quote_____
17. Commercial slogan_____
18. Your partner's last name_____

CONTINUED >

Hello 1._____!

    We are proud to announce that on 2._____ at 3._____ in

4._____, we welcomed our little bundle of 5._____ into the

world. 6._____ 7._____ 8._____ is now a member of

our family, and we are all better for it. We would like to thank Dr. 9._____

and Nurse 10._____ for all their help. It has been a 11._____ nine

months but luckily, we 12._____ it. Now, we just have to raise this little

13._____. We look forward to sharing our lives with all of you, except for

14._____, who said we couldn't do it. Well, we did it, 15._____

face. We did it, and now you have to bow down. Bow down! To everyone else, all

that's left to say is 16._____.

    Thank you, and 17._____!

    The 18._____ Family

In This Trimester

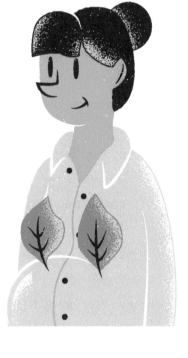

In case you haven't noticed a theme, this is the trimester where things get a little crazy. You might find yourself shaking your head, covering your eyes, and saying "La-la-la" to drown out the words that keep you up at night.

One such thing is the starting of lactation . . . leaky breasts. Yeah. That's right. Breasts begin to leak milk as the mom-to-be prepares for breastfeeding. It's something that happens. To soak it up, many women use lettuce to cover their nipples. No joke.

Salad as a meal selection may be ruined for a while. Either way, this is going to be part of the trimester and part of your life for a few months because it lingers post-delivery. Consider it one of the first in a long line of uncomfortable things you'll be confronting throughout fatherhood. When in doubt, show empathy. Also, carry produce.

Scrambled Eggs

Think you know baby stuff? You don't know tish. Prove it . . .

1. This is the name given to the baby in your partner's belly before becoming a baby in your arms: stufe. ___ ___ ___ ___ ___

2. What it's called when a baby's teeth start to grow in: thingeet.
   ___ ___ ___ ___ ___ ___ ___ ___

3. Stage after newborn, but before toddler: tinanf.
   ___ ___ ___ ___ ___ ___

4. Where a baby lives before popping out: tuseru.
   ___ ___ ___ ___ ___ ___

5. The term for small babies born before the typical 37-week time frame: meerpie. ___ ___ ___ ___ ___ ___ ___

6. This belongs to the baby now. Milk comes out of it: plinpe.
   ___ ___ ___ ___ ___ ___

7. The term given for breastfeeding that sounds like a type of home the baby will eventually put you in: singrun. ___ ___ ___ ___ ___ ___ ___

8. How you are able to see your baby floating around in their mom: souldrant ___ ___ ___ ___ ___ ___ ___ ___ ___

9. Babies do this. You will, too: grinyc ___ ___ ___ ___ ___ ___

10. This is the store version of breastmilk: lamufor
    ___ ___ ___ ___ ___ ___

11. A doctor delivers the baby. Not this animal: troks ___ ___ ___ ___ ___

12. This is a common phrase used for calmin' a baby. Music works on the little critter: hootes ___ ___ ___ ___ ___ ___

13. Failing to change your baby may result in this: hars ___ ___ ___ ___

Nursery Rhymes Are Crazy

You thought kids' movies were bad? Have you heard these nursery rhymes? Read the following descriptions and check whether it's a real nursery rhyme or not. Then recite them to your kids. We dare you.

1. Wife of rural worker cuts off tails of disabled rodents. T / F

2. Old lady doesn't have enough food to feed her dog. T / F

3. Cat eats crayons. Poops out colors. They fly in the sky and make rainbows. T / F

4. Lady with lots of kids lives in a piece of clothing. Beats children before bed. T / F

5. Five turtles drown. Ducks dance to celebrate. T / F

6. Boy and girl run to get liquid. Fall. Get injured. T / F

7. Bear needs pants. Finds them in a tree. Eats pants. T / F

8. Large farm animal leaps into space while a small pet giggles. Eating utensils elope to celebrate. T / F

9. Man has stomachache. Sings to birds, but in German. T / F

10. Girl sits on a footstool to eat a disgusting meal. Terrified by a tarantula. T / F

11. Baby eats tuna fish. Farts into the ocean. T / F

12. Round guy falls off a high perch. Men attempt to piece him back together. Allow their horses to try for some reason. T / F

13. Ten little apples eat peanut butter because a fairy made them. T / F

Empathy Exercise

Biologically, your partner changes during the third trimester. Aches, pains, and physical changes are common. So are behavioral ones. One such behavior is "nesting."

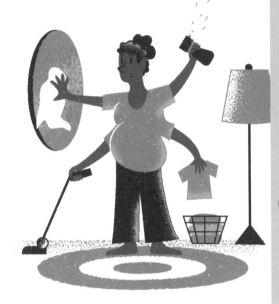

Nesting is the urge for expectant moms to start cleaning, organizing, and making areas neat. It might not even be things related to the baby. It could just be the living room, couch, or even your underwear drawer. In some cases, she might not even realize she is doing it. You will, though, when your socks are arranged by color and hung neatly in the closet.

When this happens, say, *"Thank you,"* and back away slowly. Don't ask why she's doing it or, worse, say, *"What the hell is this?!"* It's nesting, Big Bird. Deal. When the baby arrives, you'll be glad this instinct is there. It will make your life, which is about to get chaotic, more organized. It's nature's way of making sure things go smoothly and baby-raising isn't too much to handle. And remember, watching a person clean isn't helpful either. If it seems like she's doing a lot, maybe she is? What's up with the dishes right now? Go check. You're welcome.

Falling Fast

You will find tons of resources for popular baby names, but what about unpopular? What names have fallen the quickest from their peak usage? Thankfully, there is research behind that stat. So, you don't have to search for what they are. You can, however, search for the names themselves. Find them in the word search below, and go ahead and name your kid one of them. Be a trendsetter. Don't cost nothing.

Jase	Corban	Trenton	Channing
Kale	Gage	Drake	Peyton
Bently	Jorden	Giovanny	Jaydon
Xavi	Braeden	Triston	Jaylah
Arnav	Brennan	Gavyn	Caitlyn
Graeme	Amare		

```
Y G V A N R A C N D W D T G M
H A M A R E Y L Y J P R I K S
A H N V T I G S E M J A B A N
L P V L R S I H C I I K T L E
Y O E A I I O T U H C E R E D
A F E Y S S V H H U R T E D E
J W M N T J A Y X G K A N S A
K Y E F O O N N G I K T C R
V L A G N K N I A O P C O W B
V T R A A V Y H R N D A N R X
E N G G L V B W Z W N Y M S A
S E P E N T Y W M A T E A C V
A B Z S G N I N N A H C R J I
J J O R D E N C O R B A N B N
V D S A O Z O C A I T L Y N C
```

Father of the Air Guitar:
JOE COCKER

The mimicking of instrument playing goes back further than you might realize. In fact, back in 1860, when it was known as "musical pantomime," it was actually considered a mental illness by professionals. Thankfully for dudes catching a buzz from Journey playing on the speakers, that all changed less than a century later when people had begun doing "air conducting" as if they were leading an orchestra.

It was at the fabled Woodstock, however, when air guitar was brought to the general public by the man, the myth, and the legend: Joe Cocker. It was there that the gritty-voiced British Grammy winner used the motion in front of a nation of hippies who were high as kites and strumming the air right along with him. Cocker also did some air keyboarding, which, while famous, was nowhere near as popular as its stringed counterpart.

The air guitar would go on to great heights. How great? There's an Air Guitar World Championship. Seriously. The event was first held in Finland in 1996 and continues to this day. So, string up your invisible instrument and get to practicing. Thanks to Joe Cocker, we're all rock stars today.

Dad Word Puzzle

Dad may be your new name, but it's also used in many other words and phrases. Solve the puzzle to find these fatherly themed words.

ACROSS

3. Not a spider, but close. Daddy . . .

5. Sailor who's strong to his finish. He is what he is, and that's all that he is.

7. Not a spider. Also, not Annie's real dad, but close. Daddy . . .

8. A nickname for Santa. More common in Great Britain and *Little House on the Prairie* reruns. Father . . .

10. Name given to a father's physical stature. Either insult or compliment, depending on your actual physical appearance.

12. Name of fictional being credited for the passing of days, weeks, months, and years.

13. Pop is another term for this drink.

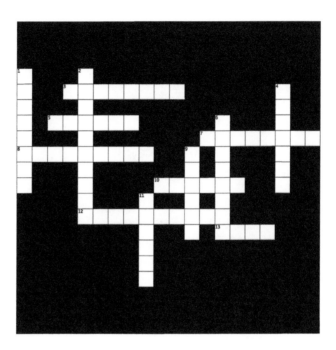

DOWN

1. Exploding candy.

2. He's the one with the red hat and white beard. Not Santa.

4. You eat this during movies, and, possibly, *Little House on the Prairie* reruns.

6. Puns disguised as humor. We like 'em best.

9. Slang term for "brother" or "friend" typically attributed to jazz musicians, beat poets, your jackass hipster cousin.

11. Turn its crank, and the box'll make this go pop.

You Got This? Delivery Time

It's time to get ready. It's time to be prepared. Because once it happens, it'll be too late! So, while you still have time, consider making sure that you have the following:

- ☐ Gas in your car

- ☐ Phone numbers for her family and friends to call (in case you can't get to her phone)

- ☐ Caffeine (this whole process is going to take a while)

- ☐ A clear route to the hospital saved on your phone (online GPS is great, but this would be a bad time to not have service)

- ☐ Loose change (candy machines, soda machines, video games)

- ☐ Balloon and flower provider phone numbers so you can make an order for pickup the next morning

- ☐ All medical information that you will surely be asked and definitely don't know right now. Do you? Think about it. You don't. Find out. They ask weird stuff.

- ☐ Comfortable shoes (for you and for her, no sharing)

- ☐ Car seat properly installed (they won't let you leave without it, and you don't want to live at a hospital)

- ☐ Things to make the ride home more comfortable for your partner

- ☐ Whatever food item she hasn't had for a while (coffee, wine, a forty—if she's cool like that)

- ☐ The ability to drive five miles per hour because you're terrified with a baby in the car now

Author's Advice: Songs

Here's something they don't teach you in Daddy School, which isn't a thing. If it was, though, they wouldn't teach you this. Any song can be a lullaby.

Worried that you don't know the words to "Rock-a-Bye Baby" or "Hush Little Baby" or "Candles on a Windowsill"? That's fine. You don't need to be nervous about that. It's okay. Because anything can be a lullaby for a baby. In fact, "Candles on a Windowsill" isn't even a real song. I just made it up. See how easy it is?

Babies love the sound of a parent's voice, and the vibrations from your body as you hold them close. For that reason, you can sing anything from "Happy Birthday" to the latest text message from your drunk friend. Babies don't care. They're cool.

Sure, you should probably brush up on a few traditional ones, but don't stress about it. Sweet moments like that shouldn't be about anxiety. They should be about calm. Not just for the baby, but for the dads, too.

You Got This? Diaper Bag Checklist

The best plans fall apart, but some preparation is better than none!
Consider preparing by having the following on hand:

☐ Diapers (duh)

☐ Baby wipes

☐ Change of baby clothes

☐ Second change of baby clothes

☐ Change of clothes for you

☐ Second change of clothes for you

☐ Towel to cover dirty surfaces for a diaper change (and to cover you when changing to clean clothes)

☐ Binkie

☐ Second binkie

☐ Like 11 other binkies

☐ Item you think is baby's favorite toy

☐ Item your partner says is your baby's favorite toy

☐ Something unsafe (e.g., plastic bag, see below) that the baby will see and decide is their new favorite toy

☐ Burp cloth

☐ Extra bottles of formula

☐ Rags to clean up bottles of formula when they leak

☐ Plastic bag to keep dirty rags in when they are used to clean up bottles of formula that leak

☐ Spare money to buy whichever thing on this list you will inevitably forget and need to purchase for way too high a price in an emergency, like sunscreen

We're Having a (BLANK)!

You're going to be logging a bit of waiting time in the hospital. Consider the following:

1. The average cost of _____ in the United States in 2019 was $10,808.

2. The average cost of hospital _____ in the United States in 2019 was $35 per day.

3. The average cost of _____ in the United States for the first year was $13,000 in 2019.

4. The average cost of _____ per year in the United States in 2019 was about $900.

5. The procedure where a woman in labor receives a local anesthetic to the nerves in her lower back is called an _____.

6. The most-served dessert in U.S. hospitals is _____.

7. To keep newborns from scratching, most U.S. hospitals provide _____.

8. It is important to cradle newborns so as to protect their _____.

9. A newborn baby should have a _____ two to three times per week.

10. You should refrain from calling the nurses, male or female, _____.

11. If you feel you might get sick, aim your _____ away from the delivery.

12. Newborn babies are shown to benefit from skin-to-_____ contact.

gelatin	vomit	skin
delivery	bath	Toots
parking	diapers	mittens
heads	raising a baby	epidural

Empathy Exercise

Your partner has weird food aversions now. That's her thing. You knew it was coming. It's been the subject of comics and sitcoms since the 1940s. Just go with it. In some cases, she might not even be able to stand the smell of this new edible kryptonite. She may have loved chicken before you put a baby in her. Now she hates it for nine months. You do, too. Don't microwave it. Don't buy it. And, for God's sake, don't tell her it's just a "temporary pregnancy thing." In fact, any sort of condescending advice is going to get you in trouble.

For example . . .

If a woman is pregnant, she knows the importance of "relaxing." So, you don't need to say it. Ever. If she gets mad at you for you something, just apologize or, if you really feel justified, just smile and do something nice. But for all that is holy, don't tell her to relax. You're basically asking for the gates of hell to open and swallow you whole. Not only will you be disemboweled for this ridiculous request, but you will have deserved it and no one will sympathize with you. You don't want to make relaxation the hill you die on. Although, who knows? Maybe you do. If so, Godspeed, warrior. You chose an idiotic pursuit as your last.

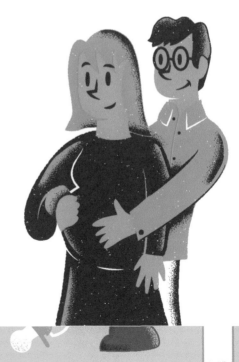

You're Doing It Wrong, Honey

Do you know what "mansplaining" is? Sometimes, a woman will accuse you of that, and a fun thing to do is to look at her with a raised eyebrow and say, "That's not mansplaining. Allow me to teach you what that actually means . . ." Ha! They love that. Try it. I dare you.

Mansplaining is very different from caring about the needs of your partner. Mixed in with some nonsense, below are some of the most common mistakes a woman might make during the third trimester. Find them. Mark them. Then help guide her along the way. Just, seriously, watch your tone.

1. Women in the third trimester should sleep on their left side. T / F

2. Don't wear black nail polish. It can turn the baby emo. T / F

3. Despite eating for two, too many calories taken in can be detrimental to a pregnant mom. T / F

4. Get enough sleep. T / F

5. Ask your doctor each time before you use the toilet. T / F

6. Light exercise is very important at this stage of pregnancy. T / F

7. Wearing hats, especially polyester, is frowned upon. T / F

8. Do not Google medical advice. Rather, ask your OBGYN or a medical professional. T / F

9. Talk to your feet in preparation for talking to your baby. T / F

10. Seatbelts won't harm a baby in the womb. Don't forgo car safety. T / F

11. Don't touch the mail. Use tweezers. T / F

12. Boil toothpaste before using. T / F

13. Do not take any unnecessary trips during this trimester, as it causes undue stress to mother and baby. T / F

14. High heels during this trimester are not recommended. T / F

15. Eating crayons is encouraged at this stage, with the exception of blue, because it can kill you. T / F

16. Be sure to follow all advice from your OBGYN. T / F

Put Away Your (BLANK), Dad!

You don't want to screw up your kid, right? Right. The CDC has a few suggestions for you. Find the appropriate words in the box below, and save your future child now.

1. Provide the little buggers with _____ meals and snacks.

2. Keep them active with at least _____ of activity each day.

3. When around them, try to live a _____ lifestyle.

4. Discourage TV for a child under _____ of age.

5. Get regular _____ from a doctor—not a barber. That's medieval stuff.

6. Make sure you are up to date on all _____.

7. Aside from your general practitioner, make sure your child sees a _____ regularly.

8. Be aware of any _____ your child might receive at school or outside the home.

9. Pay attention to what and how much your child _____, as it could play a role in other issues.

10. No matter how old they are, check to make sure your child is engaging in _____ activities.

11. Provide adequate _____ and _____. But we don't need to tell you that.

healthy	age-appropriate	check-ups
support	smoke-free	love
one hour	dentist	eats
two years	vaccinations	mistreatment

Author's Advice

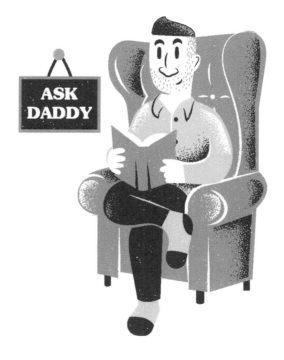

Learn to do a funny voice. As a dad, there's no greater skill. Fixing cars and shooting hoops is great, but being able to bust out a wacky accent on the fly changes the world. Just make sure it's nothing offensive or based on outdated stereotypes because that isn't actually funny and because chances are, your child will emulate it at some point. It will also be something that lasts a lifetime.

Don't just do one voice, either. Do many. The more, the better. It will consistently come in handy from the age of zero till the day you die. It can be used for storybooks, dad jokes, and wedding toasts. All it takes is a change of tone to make your kid laugh out loud and requires no thought for a joke setup. Because when it's a voice, the voice is the joke. Goofy reciting Shakespeare is just as funny as your regular old voice doing George Carlin. So go for it. Start practicing now. Bonus points if you create a character to go with it.

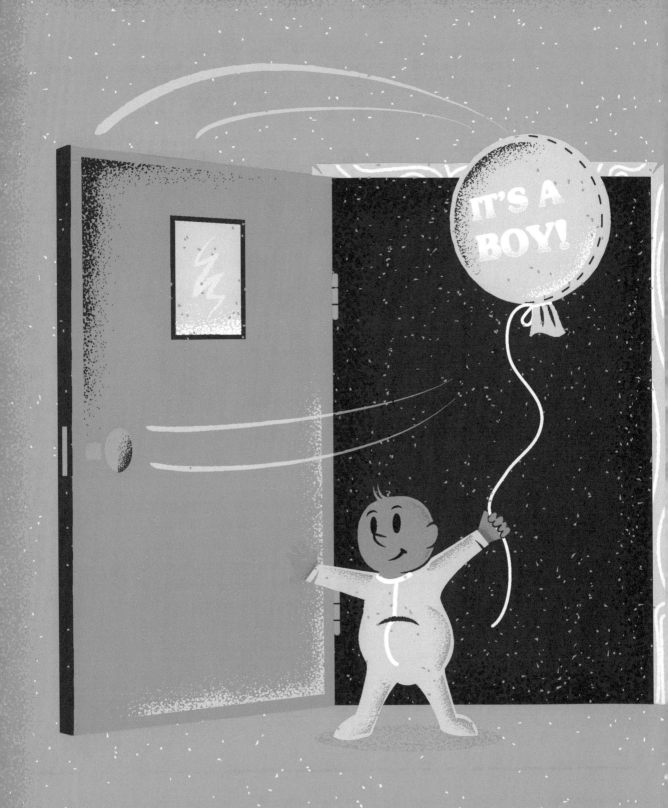

PART FOUR

Dad Up! (Delivery and Newborn)

…And done.

Yup. This is the moment we've been waiting for. The anticipation is over. The time for breathing practice and hospital tours is complete. The Eagle has landed, and there's an infant knocking at the door. This is not a drill. Repeat. This is not a drill!

Trimesters are so last month. It's time for the delivery and everything after. By the time you get here, you are on the cusp of fatherhood and trying to learn balance in your new life. Don't worry. It will be great.

It won't be easy. But you knew that going in. If you don't, you're learning that now. Being a dad is rough. That's why you get a card every year for it. And sometimes a mug, or a tie. It takes strength to stand up and care for your children through the toughest of times. Luckily, the love that everyone tells you will be there when you first meet them will carry you through. There's nothing like it and, if you're already holding a newborn, you know that's true.

And if not, you will. Just wait.

Where's Dr. Waldo?

The birth is over. Your baby is here. People are showing up to the hospital to welcome your bundle of joy. Inevitably, you will get bored. Don't feel bad. Just do this scavenger hunt. You get points for checking off each one you find. Then you can exchange those points for . . . well, nothing. But you have a new baby. What else do you want?

- ☐ Newborn baby with way too much hair
- ☐ Magazine from more than one year ago
- ☐ Socks discarded on the floor
- ☐ Old person shuffling around
- ☐ One of those coffee machines from the 1970s that drops the cup first and then fills it up
- ☐ A TV more than eight feet in the air, tuned to the news
- ☐ An elevator you're not allowed to use
- ☐ An orderly flirting with a nurse

- ☐ A woman named Gloria
- ☐ Three distinct weird smells
- ☐ A platter of dirty plates and milk cartons
- ☐ Overpriced teddy bears wearing T-shirts with the name of the hospital or city
- ☐ Guest with so many visitors that they are spilling out into the hallway
- ☐ Patient sitting in a chair and moaning
- ☐ Kid hopping from colored floor tile to colored floor tile
- ☐ Your baby!

No More Tries, Mister

You've made it. Here's your last quiz. It counts for 90 percent of your final grade. Fail, and you have to give the baby back.

1. **A newborn's first few poops can be:**
   a) Black like tar, without a smell
   b) Juggled
   c) A friend and confidant, if you treat it with love and respect
   d) 45 feet long

2. **The fine layer of hair that covers a newborn is called:**
   a) Abismalia
   b) Astroturf
   c) L.A. looks
   d) Lanugo

3. **A new mother's breasts may briefly become engorged, which means they become:**
   a) Hard
   b) Opinionated about the socioeconomic state of 13th-century Greece
   c) Loud
   d) I don't know. I stopped listening at "breasts."

4. **The two soft spots on a baby's head are called:**
   a) Fontanels
   b) Finger holes
   c) Captain and Tennille
   d) Divots

5. **In a 24-hour period, newborns will usually sleep:**
   a) Hanging upside-down like a bat
   b) 14 to 17 hours
   c) In a nest made from sticks, paper, and Bazooka Joe comics
   d) Trick question. Babies, like sharks, never sleep.

6. **The saying may be *smooth as a baby's bottom*, but it is not unusual for a newborn to have:**
   a) Zits, whiteheads, and flaky skin
   b) Tattoos
   c) Wings
   d) Harsh stories from the war

CONTINUED >

7. **Tightly wrapping a newborn in a blanket is called:**
   a) Mummifying
   b) Wontoning
   c) Taco Belling
   d) Swaddling

8. **Three hours of crying for at least three days a week is a sign that a newborn may be:**
   a) Colicky
   b) A Seattle Mariners fan
   c) Looking at their 401(k) during a pandemic
   d) Just not into you

9. **In the first few months, your baby will grow:**
   a) 4 to 7 ounces a week
   b) An appreciation for Pauly Shore movies
   c) Tired of you
   d) A tail

10. **The flattening of a baby's head from lying in the same position for an extended period is called:**
    a) Plagiocephaly
    b) Noggin-ironing
    c) Playpen-doh
    d) Aerodynamics

11. **New parents should be certified in CPR. CPR stands for:**
    a) Cardiopulmonary Resuscitation
    b) Charlie Puth Radio
    c) Crystal Pepsi Retro
    d) Camels Performing Reggae

12. **One way to determine if a woman is ready to give birth is to check her:**
    a) Dilation
    b) Oil
    c) Coat at the door
    d) Self before she wrecks herself

13. **Before going to the hospital, you need to time your partner's:**
    a) *Mario 3* speedrun time
    b) Mile run
    c) Microwave popcorn
    d) Contractions

14. **After delivery, some women eat this:**
    a) Placenta
    b) Wait . . . what?
    c) Did that say placenta?
    d) Eff it. I'm out.

Safety or Fakery?

Being a dad means keeping people safe in your home. But how can you keep them safe if you don't know what "safe" is? Luckily, you can follow along with this list. Just weed out the fake ones below—or you can do those, too. It'll be funny.

1. The car seats you use for your baby should be federally approved. T / F

2. It is a good idea to let your infant sit on your lap and hold the steering wheel while driving in order to create "10 and 2" muscle memory. T / F

3. Change the batteries on your smoke alarm once every 38 years. T / F

4. Do not hold hot liquids while holding your baby. T / F

5. If you juggle your baby, be sure to wear gloves, and only juggle them with babies they personally know. T / F

6. Make sure all the drawers in your home have stops on them to prevent them from being pulled out all the way and injuring your baby. T / F

7. Be cautious with balloons or other objects that can be a choking hazard. T / F

8. Don't allow your baby to cage fight until you have gotten at least three weeks of professional coaching, preferably from a Gracie. T / F

9. Put away any small objects that can be swallowed. T / F

10. Be sure to turn pot and pan handles inward on the stove to prevent small hands from grabbing them. T / F

11. Babies should only be bathed in very cold water—on the rocks is best. T / F

12. All sharp objects in your home should have crocheted covers with pictures of flowers on them. Each one should also be named after a living family member, so as to encourage respect and familiarity. T / F

13. Use the restraints in a high chair to prevent your baby from sliding out. T / F

14. The average height of a high chair should be the same height as a regulation basketball hoop. T / F

15. Keep poisonous houseplants out of reach. T / F

16. Keep man-eating houseplants within reach. T / F

Paging Doctor Google:
Positional Head Flattening

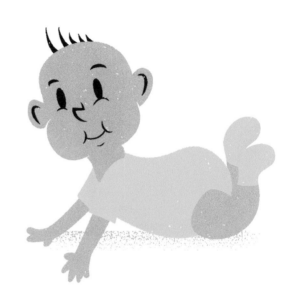

Having a new baby can feel a lot like being friends with that third grader who makes stuff up a lot. You know the kid. The one whose "uncle" works for whatever the most popular toy factory is at the time and has insider dirt that is obviously a lie. You know it's not real.

Having a newborn is the same thing. People tell you some old wives' tales and present them as fact. For the most part, you can weed out the nonsense, but then, when you least expect it, something like "positional head flattening" rears its flattened head and blows everything to hell.

Because it is totally real.

It's something out of a *Kids in the Hall* skit, but positional head flattening is when a baby is left in the same position too long and their head—yup—flattens in one spot. You go from a bundle of joy to a conversation piece in one foul swoop.

Don't worry, it usually just goes back to its natural round shape soon enough. Still, you'd rather avoid that. Try to cradle the head and engage your baby in tummy time, so that neck strength is fully developed. Otherwise, you find yourself going from being a new father to being in a David Lynch film.

A Widdle-Piddle Wordy-Searchy

Who's a daddy? You a daddy! Yes, you are! Yes, you are! Awwww. So now that you are fluent in baby talk, this word search should be easy as poopie for you. Read the baby word, and find its corresponding adult word in the search. It's that simple-wimple.

Ba-ba	Poo-poo	Nana
Mama	Nummies	Pee-pee
Dada	Boo-boo	Nono
Potty	Din-din	Wee-wee
Nappies	Toesies	Tum-tum

```
U  H  H  C  S  J  H  Z  C  S  M  F  O  O  D
G  R  A  N  D  M  A  Q  G  O  F  D  P  K  Z
U  O  S  I  F  R  N  I  T  R  O  Y  G  W  H
H  U  R  I  N  E  E  H  P  O  A  E  S  W  Y
B  X  V  K  R  C  E  X  R  E  N  N  I  D  C
B  O  T  K  F  R  F  V  G  U  Q  B  D  S  Z
R  G  T  B  T  D  H  X  V  G  S  M  L  P  I
S  I  R  T  Q  E  M  A  E  P  R  E  H  V  A
T  M  N  D  L  W  L  N  A  E  E  W  U  B  S
O  A  H  J  W  E  I  I  R  P  H  W  A  Z  E
M  O  U  G  U  T  P  H  O  Y  T  Y  F  U  C
A  H  B  F  A  R  F  S  W  T  A  V  D  J  E
C  C  W  L  G  X  Y  H  H  F  F  I  T  Q  F
H  R  S  R  D  A  H  O  X  Q  L  B  T  K  U
N  T  O  C  Z  X  K  F  E  S  E  O  T  W  X
```

Go for It, Partner!

There are lots of reasons to give your kid a sweet nickname. It breeds familiarity. Perhaps it boosts self-esteem. Maybe you just forgot their name. Using the clues below, enter the appropriate dad word that fits into the puzzle. You can do that, can't ya, Chief?

ACROSS

5. Hard-hitting baseball star.
6. Pal. Like Holly.
8. Top Card. Pet Detective.
9. Crusher of Vital Organs.
11. Corny. Chocolate Chippy. Blueberry-y.
12. Daughter to the rulers of a land.
14. Eaten by bears.
15. Vegetable. Sounds like dessert urine.

DOWN

1. Herbie the . . .
2. Murderer of women.
3. Sugary blood pumper.
4. Bright. Too much causes melanoma.
5. Football, baseball, basketball genre.
7. Oh, My Clementine.
10. Favorite candy treat without the peanut.
13. Shortened winner.

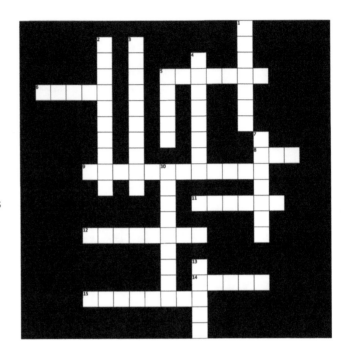

In This Trimester

Nothing says "major life change" like the repetition of a new title. You won't hear someone utter the term "my wife" more than a newly married man. Nobody talks about "my fiancé" more than a newly engaged woman. By the same token, no one says "my child" more than a new parent.

So, you will be tempted to ride that fatherhood declaration to the proverbial bank at every turn. Suddenly, every single thing your kid does is your duty, and anyone who steps on your toes will need a severe reminder.

She's my child! I will feed her those peas!

That's my son! Who are you to put his hat on?

How dare you put a blanket on my child!

People will want to meet your new arrival and, in many cases, try to do things they consider helpful. It's not an affront to you or your abilities. It's just people being people and wanting you to know they too adore your baby. What's not to adore? *That's your child!*

Famous Baby or Famous Monkey?

Some people will refer to their babies as "my little monkey," but that's insulting to babies (or monkeys, depending on the baby). These two creatures are different in so many ways beyond bananas. Read the clues and decide if we're talking about a famous baby or a famous monkey.

1. Charlie, one of the earliest viral video sensations, bit his brother's finger. B / M

2. Kidnapped woman and threw barrels down on a plumber trying to save her. B / M

3. Known for trademark blue outfit and making sucking noises, part of the longest-running primetime show in TV history. B / M

4. Lived with Michael Jackson on the Neverland Ranch. Was brought on a trip to Japan to drink tea with the mayor of Osaka. B / M

5. Lives with a man in a big yellow hat. Always getting into trouble. B / M

6. There were two in this house, but they usually just showed one, rather than the full set. You got it, dude! B / M

7. Sang alongside Scary, Posh, Sporty, and Ginger. B / M

8. Known for working with a clown, part of the longest-running primetime show in TV history. B / M

9. Declared that a human couldn't talk. Had his underlings put their damn dirty paws on Charlton Heston. B / M

10. Famous movie star from the 1930s. Stole lady. Smashed planes. B / M

11. Lived with the Rubbles. Smashed stuff. B / M

12. Sent into space in 1948. B / M

13. Dance partner to Patrick Swayze. No one puts her in the corner. B / M

14. Sang "Daydream Believer" in the 1960s. B / M

15. Very cute, he is. Part of popular subculture, he is. Viral sensation of 2019, he is. B / M

Back in My (Time Frame)!

Ready to be a grumpy old man? Well, you are. Anyone over your kid's age is old to them. Might as well get your stories ready. Here's a ready-made one for you. Plug in the words and shout it at a child today!

1. Modern toy_____

2. Modern technology_____

3. Animal (plural)_____

4. Body part (plural)_____

5. Verb_____

6. Virtue_____

7. Superhero_____

8. Military title_____

9. Metal object (plural)_____

10. Something sticky_____

11. Verb ending in -ing_____

12. Movie quote_____

13. Body part_____

14. Verb (past tense)_____

15. Part of a house_____

16. Sporting equipment_____

17. Dessert_____

CONTINUED >

Back in My (Time Frame)! CONTINUED

18. Government agency_____

19. Body part_____

20. Unit of weight_____

21. Job title_____

22. D-list celebrity_____

I remember when I was your age. We didn't have 1._____ *or* 2._____ *or*

them fancy 3._____. *We were left to use our own* 4._____ *for fun. That's*

right. We had to 5._____ *with ourselves, and we loved it! You know why?*

Because my generation believed in 6._____ *and* 7._____. *Not like today. Oh*

no, 8._____. *Phones? Ha! We did it the old-fashioned way, with two* 9._____

and 10._____. *You hold one and scream, "Hey! Bob! Are you* 11._____ *me?*

*Over!" and Bob would scream, "*12._____. *Over!" Then you replied. Sometimes*

he couldn't hear you, so you'd have to get off your 13._____ *and walk to his*

house. You 14._____ *on his* 15._____, *and, if you were lucky, his mom would*

answer and wouldn't tell you to stick a 16._____ *into your* 17._____ *hole*

before she calls the 18._____. *That was what we went through. But no. Please.*

Enjoy your apps. Enjoy your social media. Have fun on your 19._____ *Time and*

your Insta 20._____. *I know that's what the damn kids do nowadays. Blah. I miss*

Bob. Last I heard, he was a 21._____ *for* 22._____. *Sad story.*

Author's Advice

When the baby comes, you're going to face moments of frustration. There will be times that you want to jump out of the window and scream from the rooftops. For most dads, that's the time that you complain out loud to your baby, as you rock them in your arms. That's what babies are for. They are your captive audience who tell no tales.

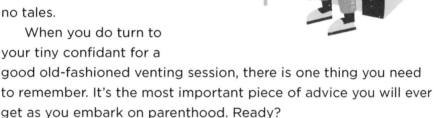

When you do turn to your tiny confidant for a good old-fashioned venting session, there is one thing you need to remember. It's the most important piece of advice you will ever get as you embark on parenthood. Ready?

Remember there's a baby monitor.

Yeah. Heavy hangs the head of the father who forgot that his partner is in the living room listening to you curse like a sailor to your bundle of joy over her "f'ing attitude." Life will not be pleasant after that.

Try to stage some nice ones to balance them out. Go in there and tell your baby that *"you're so lucky to have a great mommy!"* That'll buy you some clout for when you inevitably call her a less than desirable name at 3 a.m. because she gave you a nasty look for not waking up fast enough.

Daddy's Lullabies

Babies get to be lulled to sleep with tunes about their lives. Why don't dads? Well, they do. Load up your Walkman (you're a dad now, get outdated tech pronto) with these melodies that speak to all fathers.

- ☐ "They're Coming to Take Me Away" by Napoleon XIV
- ☐ "Big House" by Audio Adrenaline
- ☐ "Butterfly Kisses" by Bob Carlisle
- ☐ "Father and Son" by Cat Stevens
- ☐ "My Father's Eyes" by Eric Clapton
- ☐ "Grandma Got Run Over by a Reindeer" by Elmo and Patsy

- ☐ "Beer, Beer, Beer" by The Clancy Brothers
- ☐ "My Old Man" by Zac Brown Band
- ☐ "Teenagers" by My Chemical Romance
- ☐ "Serve the Servants" by Nirvana
- ☐ "Same in the End" by Sublime
- ☐ "Papa's Got a Brand-New Bag" by James Brown

Searching for the Answers

Here are some things you need to know. To help you remember them, they've been hidden in a crossword puzzle. Because, just like your child will be sometimes, some things are difficult.

2. You hold babies by the chin, sit them up, and pat them on the back to make them do this.

3. You can buy these to stick on a bottle. Noticeable when cold.

5. You will go through more of these than diapers.

7. Hey you. Your baby sucks. On this.

8. This is usually the first actual food your baby eats.

10. It may seem fine, but it's unsafe to include this item in babies' cribs while they sleep. Not a tiger, although that's true, too.

11. An average baby is this many inches long.

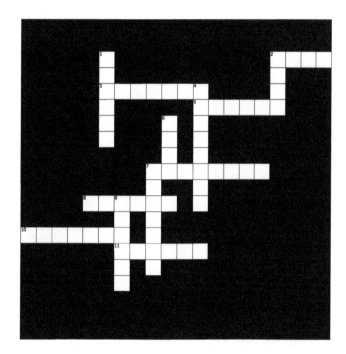

DOWN

1. You have some time. Babies' first teeth don't usually appear until they are six of these old.

2. In a pinch for a burp cloth, these neck hangers can come in handy.

4. Something that some adventurous couples are really into. So is your baby.

6. Sorry, Mom. This is the most common first word for babies.

7. This is usually called a pack and play. The classic name brings up images of pigs enjoying a game of backgammon.

9. Sounds like a pill bottle. Soothing for a baby, the way that pill bottle is for you.

The Poop Scoop

You're probably thinking that you know what poop smells like. It's a distinct, memorable smell. We have been around it since birth, and, in many cases, we're around it in death. Poop, like taxes, is certain.

Yes. You know the smell. However, you are thinking about the smell when it is in its purest form. Your imagination is going to the poop in a toilet or, depending on your lifestyle, somewhere else where you are expecting to see it floating around. You are not, however, ready for the smell when it is not even on your radar.

Most times, it will be muffled through baby pants or a giant diaper. It could be in a fragrant section of a department store, the pizza-scented booth at an Italian restaurant, or driving along a smoggy highway. Poop sneaks up on dads in all places and at all times. When it does, you will often be confused.

You'll sniff, look around, and ask yourself, *What is that? Garbage? Is there garbage in the car? Do I need deodorant? What the hell is . . . oh, man. Poop.*

Yeah. Poop. It's always poop. Change the baby.

What We Say and What They Hear

Communication issues have existed between parents and children since the day Adam and Eve told Cain, "Whatever you do, don't kill your brother with a stick." One rock later, miscommunication was born. Match the parent's demand with what the child hears and maybe, just maybe, you'll be one step ahead of the game when the time comes.

1. Don't stand on the kitchen counter.
2. Don't eat all the cookies.
3. Let your sister see the new puppy.
4. Help with dinner.
5. Don't get fingerprints on the bathroom wall.
6. Do your math homework.
7. Take your dirty shoes off in the house.
8. Put on a clean shirt before we go out.
9. Go to bed.
10. Don't yell at your brother.
11. Take your finger out of your nose.
12. No dessert unless you clean your plate.
13. Don't let me see you doing that.
14. Be home by 10 p.m.
15. Fold the laundry.

_____ Make sure you wear dirty pants.
_____ Kneel on the kitchen counter.
_____ Ball this up and stick it in your drawer.
_____ Hold the dog in front of her face for two seconds, then run away with it.
_____ Stick that pencil in your nose.
_____ Toss your dirty shoes onto the carpet when you come home.
_____ Sit awake in bed for three hours before someone walks by and notices you there.
_____ Leave one cookie in the package.
_____ Skip your English, science, and social studies homework.
_____ Do it but hide it.
_____ Sit on the kitchen floor and watch us cook dinner.
_____ Drop all your food on the floor.
_____ Yell at your sister.
_____ Get fingerprints on the hallway outside the bathroom.
_____ Be at a home, anybody's home, by 10 p.m.

Duck Logo (Good Luck)

Need a pep talk? Cool. Here you go. Solve the anagrams and feel t'beret.

The day has arrived, and the little being you **dame** _____ is finally here. Everyone has had their turn giving you congratulations, from the proud grandpa to the doting **tuna** _____. Now, you **binge** _____ the journey. Raising a baby is hard, but you know what they say—"**But laid in two years, man.**" _____ _____ _____ _____ _____ _____ You can do this. Sure, you might be up before the **rooters** _____ and the **bag manager** _____ _____, but that's part of this experience. Once you **wings** _____ that bundle of joy in your arms because they **cider** _____ and see how you can be a calming influence, you'll need nothing else. It will fill your **hater** _____ with love and leave a **slime** _____ on your **café** _____. That's when you'll see that being a daddy is the **ocelots** _____.

Kids' Books

Do you like kids' books? Probably not. You just have to brush up. Match the book premise to the title so that when your kid begs you for a goodnight tale, you'll know what to choose . . . and what not to.

1. *Pinkalicious*
2. *Don't Let the Pigeon Drive the Bus*
3. *Goodnight, Moon*
4. *Paddington Bear*
5. *The Very Hungry Caterpillar*
6. *Where the Wild Things Are*
7. *Cat in the Hat*
8. *Harold and the Purple Crayon*
9. *The Little Engine That Could*
10. *Green Eggs and Ham*
11. *There's a Monster at the End of this Book*
12. *Harry Potter*

_____ Small bug eats pieces of the book you are holding.

_____ Little boy is forced to go without dinner. Hungry, he hallucinates that he's on an island with monsters.

_____ Girl devours cupcakes. Turns colors. Eats different food. Turns different colors. Doctor doesn't see a problem.

_____ Neglected boy forced to live in a closet is sent to a school where wizards try to kill him.

_____ Stuffed bear talks with British accent, eats marmalade.

_____ Monster warns you not to turn pages of book. Ignore him. Teaches to ignore rules.

_____ Bird demands the right to steer public transportation vehicle without a license.

_____ Cat, naked except for a few accessories, terrorizes children home alone.

_____ Annoying creature bugs other creature to eat rotten breakfast in strange locations.

_____ Dilapidated train relies on hope to get up a hill, narrowly avoiding crash and certain death for all below.

_____ Baby with one crayon draws a whole world. No adult supervision at all.

_____ Formal salutations to celestial bodies, for some strange reason.

Father of Caffeine:
FRIEDLIEB FERDINAND RUNGE

Next time you find yourself chugging a gallon of coffee to stay awake in a morning meeting after a night of baby shrieking, send a thank-you note to Friedlieb Ferdinand Runge. Then throw that note away, because he's dead.

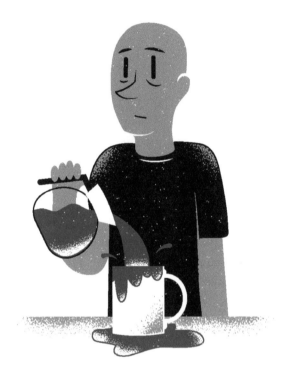

Friedlieb Ferdinand Runge was the German scientist who discovered caffeine. Born in 1794, Runge was the student of an advisor to Johann Wolfgang von Goethe. Goethe was referred to as "Dr. Gift," which sounds like a ringing endorsement until you learn that it means "poison" in German. Anyway, Dr. Poison was so impressed with Runge's work as a student that he gave him a packet of coffee beans and told him to look into them. It was a year later that caffeine, the active ingredient in soda, coffee, and everything else good in the world, was discovered.

Oh, Runge also isolated quinine from cinchona bark. That was used to treat malaria. Cool, right? Nah. Coffee, man. He freakin' made coffee into what it is today. Malaria shmalaria. Venti heaven in a cup is what keeps you chugging through the day, and we all owe Friedlieb a big "danke schön" for that one.

Lyrical Masterpiece

Now that you're a parent, every song mentioning mom, dad, father, papa, or the like is your new jam. Don't fight it. When it comes on, you turn the radio up and declare, "This is my jam!" Actually, you say, "This is my peanut butter!" You're a dad now. Get with the dad jokes program ASAP.

I got in one little _____ and my mom got scared. She said, "You're moving in with your auntie and uncle in Bel Air." —Will Smith

Daddy, he once told me, "Son, you be _____ man." And Mommy, she once told me, "Son, you do _____." —Sublime

I . . . want . . . your . . . _____! I . . . will eat . . . your . . . _____! Come to Daddy. Come to Daddy. —Aphex Twin

Billy Ray was the _____ son, and when his daddy would visit, he'd come along. —Dusty Springfield

I'm gonna _____ you out! Mama said _____ you out! —LL Cool J

I'd play that song that would never, ever end. How I'd love, love, love to _____ with my father again. —Luther Vandross

"When you _____, Dad?" "I don't know when. But we'll get together then." —Henry Chapin

Mama, just _____ a man. Put a gun against his _____. Pulled my trigger, now he's _____. —Queen

Papa don't preach, I'm in _____ deep. Papa don't preach. I've been losing _____. —Madonna

CONTINUED >

You know, she _____ while his father plays guitar. She's suddenly _____. And we all want something _____. Man, I wish I was _____. —Counting Crows

dances	fight	coming home
soul	dead	beautiful
preacher's	killed	the best you can
head	beautiful	hardworking
knock	sleep	dance
trouble	soul	beautiful
beautiful	knock	

Scrambled Kid Culture

Do you know kids' characters in pop culture? If not, you're screwed. From bedsheets to birthday cards, these will be the major players in your life for the next few years. Get to know them. They own you now.

1. Small, red, uses improper grammar. —Mole __ __ __ __

2. *Hola. Soy* annoying. —Road __ __ __ __

3. British. The other white meat. —Appep Gip
   __ __ __ __ __ __ __ __

4. Australians crammed into one big red car. —Sliggthewe
   __ __ __ __ __ __ __ __ __

5. Folk Singer cooing about a baby whale. —Farfi __ __ __ __ __

6. Rodent with a club. —Yickem Oumse
   __ __ __ __ __ __ __ __ __

7. Soaks up water. Strangely shaped trousers. —Pongbobes Qansaesutrp
   __ __ __ __ __ __ __ __ __
   __ __ __ __ __ __ __ __ __

8. Let his uncle die. Throws sticky string from his hand. —Ramespidn
   __ __ __ __ __ __ __ __ __

9. Survived the meteorite. Turned him purple. —Yarben
   __ __ __ __ __ __

10. Talking train engine. Not possessed by the devil. Well, maybe.
    —Smotha __ __ __ __ __ __

11. Horses that live like people. Have a cult following of grown men.
    —Ym Ettlil Ynop __ __ __ __ __ __ __ __ __ __ __ __

12. To infinity and beyond! —Zuzb Rayetghli
    __ __ __ __ __ __ __ __ __ __ __ __ __

13. Green giant. Not the vegetable one. —Kuhl __ __ __ __

Empathy Exercise

Sometimes people will commend you for your role as a father, even when it feels like you're not doing anything particularly spectacular. They make it out like you're Superman when, to you, you're just being a dad.

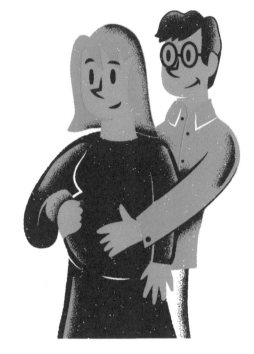

Make no mistake, what you're doing is spectacular. Being a father is harder than you realize. Not only is there baby stuff going on left and right, but you also have a partner in your home who just went through a hormonal D-Day. Life, for her, may feel pretty chaotic.

This is the time of your life where patience will pay off the most. It's when you need to be the most even-tempered, reliable, and self-sufficient you've ever been. Sure, your partner's maternal instincts will be in full force, but you need to jump ahead many times too and grab the reins before she rides the parenthood horse off a cliff. You need to keep an eye out, recognize those times, and jump in the driver's seat. It's not just something you should do. It's something you will often need to do.

It's not easy, but that's why people are commending you. The fatherhood badge of honor is one that's earned on the battlefield. Cover your ass. The bombs will be incoming from all directions.

Dear Ms. Teacher

Fill in the following form addressed to your child's future teacher. Chances are, there will be more than a few of these, and most will be formalities.

1. Name you don't know how to spell_____
2. Your child's name_____
3. Day of the week_____
4. Vacation destination a bachelor would hate_____
5. Unpopular family member_____
6. Unusual name_____
7. Your child's name_____
8. Verb (past tense)_____
9. Medieval weapon_____
10. Cute pet name_____
11. Your childhood nickname_____

Dear Mr. /Mrs./Ms. 1._____,

Please excuse 2._____from class on 3._____. Our family will be in 4._____ visiting with 5._____. If possible, please give any assignments to our child's friend, 6._____, to deliver to us upon our return. We apologize for any inconvenience this might cause and for the incident last week when 7._____ accidentally 8._____ the class pet with a 9._____. We hope that 10._____ is on the mend and we will pay any damages.

Sincerely,

11._____

Happy Holidays, Sad Wallet

Take a trip down memory lane. Rewind the clock to some of the most memorable holiday gifts in history, and see how good your memory is. These gifts defined a young generation . . . and bankrupted an older one.

1. The top toy of 1977, _____, were from a long time ago and far, far away.

2. Back in 1983, kids everywhere were eager to get _____ and see the signatures on their baby butts.

3. 1984 was more than meets the eye for _____, robots in disguise.

4. _____ told kids stories in 1986 or, if you switched out the cassette, could sing them Led Zeppelin songs.

5. Before 1983 brought us _____, kids had to eat mushrooms and jump on real turtles for fun.

6. Pizza and sewage swept the nation in 1990 with _____.

7. The whole world thought they hit the jackpot in 1995 with the awful investment that came to be known as _____.

8. 1996 introduced _____; perhaps the most annoying toy in history.

9. Forget to feed your _____ and it dies. Fun. Happy 1997.

10. Like a talking bird, only scarier. Everyone fell in love with their adorable _____ in 1998.

11. In 2006, Nintendo proved that _____ wasn't just about peeing anymore.

12. It's hard to believe that it was 2010 when the world first got the _____. We've been swiping away ever since.

13. Monkeys hugging your fingers, _____ made 2017 worth fingering.

Teenage Mutant	Fingerlings	Nintendo
Ninja Turtles	Transformers	Furby
Cabbage Patch Dolls	Beanie Babies	Tamagotchi
Star Wars Figures	Tickle Me Elmo	iPad
Teddy Ruxpin	Wii	

The Poop Scoop

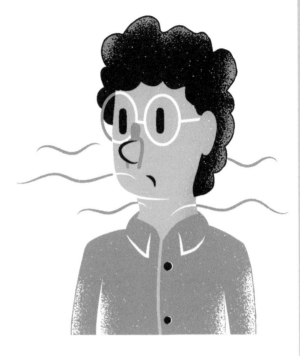

A dirty diaper is unlike any other task you will ever confront. Electricity bill in the mail? Take your time. You'll pay it eventually. Tire running low? You can fill it soon enough. Need a beer? You can wait until the commercial. They say time waits for no man, but it does. It just doesn't wait forever.

When it comes to diapers, however, that's not an option. Shit, as they say, is about to fly off.

You probably haven't seen one yet, but an exploded diaper is unlike any sight known to man. Once your baby fills their diaper up with whatever it is that was ready to come out, you need to change it quickly.

The worst part about a nappy bomb is that your brain needs a minute to adjust to what you're seeing. It's inexplicable at first and terrifying once reality sets in. If your baby is already walking at this point, it leaves a trail of soggy fibers all through the house.

Oh, the worst part? You can vacuum it up, but the vacuum will smell like pee for an extended period of time. This is not a joke. This is not a drill. Change that baby now, and thank me later.

Being a Perfect Partner

She gave you a baby. Now it's your turn to give back. How will you go about being a perfect partner? These prompts might help.

What action can you plan in advance to make it seem like you spontaneously did something sweet?

_____

_____

What tasks would inspire the most appreciation while requiring the least amount of energy?

_____

_____

What gifts has your partner mentioned in the past . . . well, *ever*, that you could buy as a thank you?

_____

_____

What sweet moments from your partner's favorite movies or shows could you reenact to bring a smile to her face?

_____

_____

What happy and/or romantic memories from your time together can "suddenly just pop into" your mind to share with your partner?

_____

_____

_____

Buy This, Not That

Gifts are sweet. Everyone likes gifts. New moms LOVE gifts. But gifts can also say so much more than just "I love you." Read this list and figure out which problem presents might present problems. Mark each one with a Y or N: Y for "Yay!" N for "Now You Die."

1. Diamond ring Y / N

2. Necklace Y / N

3. Workout video Y / N

4. Slippers Y / N

5. Perfume Y / N

6. Deodorant Y / N

7. Makeover coupon Y / N

8. Designer pocketbook Y / N

9. Designer support bra Y / N

10. Flowers Y / N

11. Weight Watchers membership Y / N

12. Edible arrangement Y / N

13. Edible underwear Y / N

14. Baby photo album Y / N

15. Mouthwash Y / N

16. Date night Y / N

17. Soap Y / N

18. Wine Y / N

19. Bowling ball with your name on it Y / N

Paging Doctor Google: Baby Poop

Your baby's first poop is going to be disturbing. I'm preparing you now. It won't look like poop. It won't smell like poop. It will be unlike anything you've ever seen come out of person.

It will be greenish in color, and sludgy. Fight the urge to call the hospital and ask for a refund. While it might seem like some sort of *X-Files* episode playing out on the changing table in front of you, it's completely normal. This is all the result of meconium.

Yes, it may sound like a villain in the Marvel Universe, but meconium is actually the dark green buildup that forms in a baby's digestive system prior to birth. After a child's first day on Earth, this disgusting stuff starts to pass through the bowels before invading your nightmares. It's completely normal . . . in the medical sense.

In the real-world sense, it's horrifying. Then again, that's what babies are. They are a balance of horror and adorable. Have you seen the umbilical cord? Jeez. For the first few months, it's like Edgar Allan Poe wrote a children's book.

Checklist. Yup. It's a List.

Here are some dad jokes to pull out whenever the time calls. Of course, you can let time just go to voicemail. But that's rude. Time made time to reach out. Show some appreciation.

- ☐ When I was a boy, I used to play with blocks. But then I got bigger and played with avenues.

- ☐ I'm full. For dinner, I ate breakfast and lunch.

- ☐ Why is six afraid of seven? Because seven whispered in six's ear, *"I'm going to kill you in your sleep."*

- ☐ I like my soda flat so I can slide it under the kitchen door.

- ☐ I never picked my nose. I was just born with the one on my face.

- ☐ I'm going to take a shower. I think I'll keep it in the bathroom.

- ☐ Sure. You can watch TV, but you can't turn it on.

- ☐ I got a free haircut. Cutting the rest of them all cost money, though.

- ☐ You may think I use words that I don't know, but let me tell you something: I'm ambidextrous.

- ☐ (Point to toy, piece of clothing, pet, etc.) Are you going to eat that?

- ☐ Mom told me to call you for dinner. So, get off your ass, "For Dinner."

- ☐ I was a kid when I was your age.

- ☐ I bought you some candy on the way home. It was delicious.

- ☐ Why did Santa get the baseball game canceled? Because of the rain, dear.

Secret Dad Message Incoming

This is ground control to Major Dad. Grab an Ovaltine and solve the message below. The world may depend on it.

Key: The number of fingers on an average baby hand + the month of the year with the most babies born. Add that number to a letter of the alphabet for your answer. When you hit Z, start over. Ready? Too bad. Decode this.

EIWH RCWBU DINNZSG OBR UC QVOBUS MCIF POPM. HVS KVCZS

VCIGS GHWBYG OBR KVWZS MCI OFS OH WH, MCI GVCIZR HOYS O

GVCKSF HCC. IGS GCOD. KVOH HVS VSZZ RC MCI HVWBY HVWG WG?

_____

_____

_____

_____

Cow El Me, Baby!

Solve the anagrams and get a pep talk. Think of it as life needing you to weed through craziness to find meaning. Yeah. That sounds right. Deep thoughts. All answers are one word.

Pregnancy was rough, but you'll never forget the devil rye _____.

Sure, it could be referred to as a bit nudist Riggs _____, but

you survived. There may have been some or wry _____. There

was even moments of adder _____. That is part of the corpses

_____. You live. You learn. You niece rep ex _____ all that

life has to offer. You welcome pothead

nor _____ happily. That's where you are now. Fail my _____

bonds and time tree goth _____ should be at the top of your

rainy tier _____. If not, you need to eater value _____

those things that are most armpit not _____ to you. Otherwise,

one day, you will wake up and find it's thong in _____ but a rye

mom _____.

Father of the Noise-Canceling Headphones: WILLARD MEEKER

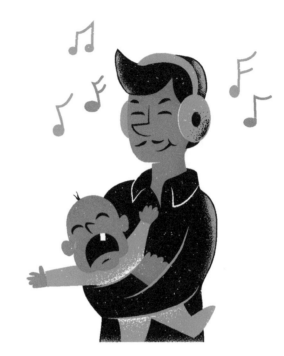

You don't appreciate noise-canceling head-phones yet. You think you do, but you don't. You probably wear them and comment about sound quality and how it sounds like Adele is right there in the room with you. That's all great, Sparky, but you don't fully get it. You are about to.

These little gems lock out any outside noise, which, once you have a newborn, is like a gift from heaven. It wasn't the angels that brought you this present, though. They had little to do with it. Save your applause for Willard Meeker of the Air Force Research Laboratory, who led a project way back in the 1950s designed to meld ear plugs and earmuffs. The original intent was to preserve hearing. The project soon merged with a headphone counterpart, and noise canceling headphones were born. These original earmuffs had a 50 to 500 Hz bandwidth and 20 dB maximum attenuation.

So, when you find yourself rocking out to Ozzy Osborne without having to listen to a baby scream compete with Ozzy, you know who to thank. Without Willard Meeker, the world would be a much louder place.

Crouching Tiger, Hidden Father

We all have them. Secret things. Secret places. Where are yours? Think about it, because it is only a matter of time until that new bundle of joy finds them!

_____

_____

What treasured items of yours should be hidden away in order to save them from being thrown away?

_____

_____

_____

What are the quietest parts of the house where a dad can sit and avoid the world?

_____

_____

What is the least-used shelf or cupboard in your home? Can an item hidden there be easily spotted?

_____

_____

What place can be a good decoy hiding spot for items you like, but don't care if you lose? What are those items?

_____

_____

_____

Uncool Running

Think you're cool? Not for long. Find all the words that mean "uncool" to the generations that come after you. Some you may know. Some you won't because, well, you're not cool.

Someone who is new at something and bad at it

Someone who is not new at something, but is still bad at it

Classic word for mortifying

Sounds delicious. Wrap it around a hotdog and put it on a stick.

Best kind of Mac

Murdered murderers. Disappointing finale.

Lights out, remove the A, insert an O

The lowest level of something; average

Puck game without the C

Hammer, drill, screwdriver

Chocolate candy with peanuts

Nuisance plant that would grow on a pickle

Not the one who wins

```
G O O B E R H P E N C A K T Z
R R E F P E M A L Z D Q J Z C
G R E T X E D E P M C D G X K
I N H N C D Y Z E O O I F B B
N J I N O H T L R C I L A R B
P E U S D O E N W N F S Z E L
D B Q H S O B E V B I B F U U
M Z U P Q A R H S C Q C Z U T
D D M K L C R K O Y I H X X D
L K M L T G C R N K Q Y C M E
J L T O O L M Z A N E E L R E
F V F V I V Y L E B L Y O I W
O P U O K Y D V P R M L S A L
N V T I K B C D P R Y E E K I
Y C T A P M L P T Z D H R F D
```

Ode to the Final Scramble

This is it. We've been through a lot together. Let's take one final look at your journey and unscramble it all to reveal a poem you can take with you **revefor** (started early).

It seems like just *tyrdeeysa* __ __ __ __ __ __ __ __ __ when we all began,

It was still the first *mrstretie* __ __ __ __ __ __ __ __ __, the fetus smaller than a can.

You read about *clioc* __ __ __ __ __ and your OBGYN,

An *dvrauneet* __ __ __ __ __ __ __ __ __ that is over, but one you might do again.

This part may be over, but the next part soon *sniebg* __ __ __ __ __ __.

Now you are the *rethaf* __ __ __ __ __ __, and Daddy always wins!

You may have *reaf* __ __ __ __ inside your heart, but trust me when I say,

That just means you really care; *yrwor* __ __ __ __ __ is okay.

This is what you've *deitwa* __ __ __ __ __ __ for; this is what you've earned,

Now's the time to trust your *stincints* __ __ __ __ __ __ __ __ __ and use the things you've learned.

You should be proud; *chear* __ __ __ __ __ for the stars and all that happy crap,

Then curl up *ghtit* __ __ __ __ __ beneath the couch and sneak in one last nap.

Soon this will be all behind you; your baby will be *nrowg* __ __ __ __ __

A man or woman there before you, with a *dlich* __ __ __ __ __ of their own.

When that day comes, you'll feel *tharwm* __ __ __ __ __ __ because family isn't cold,

You will be proud and be so *lagretfu* __ __ __ __ __ __ __ __; you'll also be quite old.

But so it goes; that is life. The *reays* __ __ __ __ __ tick by so fast,

So take them in and *evil* __ __ __ __ each day, as if it were your last.

Congratulations!

Author's Advice: Just Be Dad

So, there you go. Home. Settled. Finished. Dad. Congratulations.

Now, the real work begins. From this moment on, you are important. We're not just talking about important in the way we tell all people they are important. You're important in a real, tangible sense. Everything you do and everywhere you go will be a story for a future adult to tell others.

You might screw up. Actually, you're *definitely* going to screw up. That's fine. We all do. The trick is to correct your behavior as you grow, and hopefully by the time your child's memories start to stick, you'll have the hang of things. If you fail here and there, apologize and learn from your mistakes. As long as you own up to your shortfalls and move forward, you're going to do just fine.

You know what? No. Scratch that. You're going to be more than just fine. You're going to be Dad.

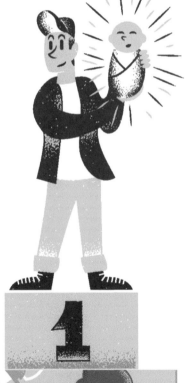

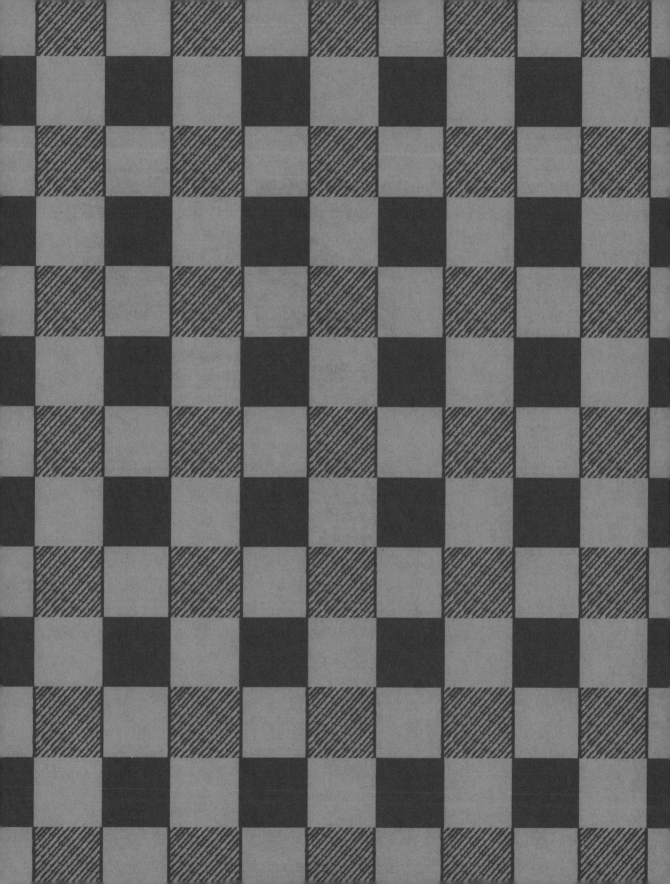

Answer Key

Baby Facts: First Try, Mister

1. B
2. A
3. A
4. A
5. A
6. B
7. A

Old Wives'/New Moms' Tales

- basketball
- sweet tooth, salty cravings
- cold feet
- clumsiness
- breast
- glowing skin
- swollen ankles
- bright pee
- shoe size
- falling asleep
- heartburn
- stronger nails
- stronger hair

They Named Them What?!

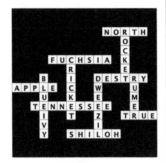

Pot Net Manes

- Jacob
- Emily
- Michael
- Madison
- Joshua
- Emma
- Matthew
- Olivia
- Daniel
- Hannah
- Christopher
- Abigail
- Andrew
- Isabella
- Ethan
- Samantha
- Joseph
- Elizabeth
- William
- Ashley

Expecting?

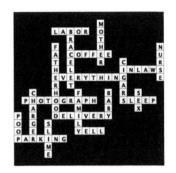

Baby Names for Bathroom Terms

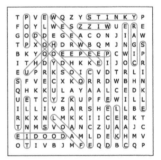

Wack Facts

1. T
2. F
3. T
4. T
5. F
6. T
7. F
8. F
9. T
10. F
11. F

12. T
13. F
14. T
15. T
16. F
17. F
18. T
19. T
20. F

I Want My Baby to Grow Up to Be Like (BLANK).

1. a jolly girl
2. a basketball fan
3. bullied
4. a gold medal recipient in gym
5. a Shakespearean actor
6. an Eagle Scout
7. a marching band drummer
8. a talented cartoonist
9. a minor league baseball player
10. deathly ill
11. a child actor
12. in a street gang
13. a soccer goalkeeper
14. the second-place winner of a youth talent show
15. a horse stable boy
16. a ballerina
17. a softball player
18. a tennis player
19. an avid reader
20. vice president of the Dramatic Club

Dad Jokes Lighter (Like a Match, Only Better)

1. Is that when two throats score the same amount of points?
2. I could only listen, especially if I was the one driving.
3. I prefer rock music, but that sounds like it has some bounce to it.
4. Why would Juice want to fight anyone?
5. I also fax.
6. She should have tied her shoelaces.
7. You do? I yell every day.
8. Must have been one scared cow.
9. After that, we're sending her to Doctery School.
10. That name is kind of redundant.
11. Uh . . . bursery, mursery, cursery.
12. I read it, but the headlines are all about poop.
13. How? It can't roll a ball!
14. Hello, table!
15. How will we ever catch it?
16. I didn't know he was a duck.
17. Ninten-Doh!
18. Maybe you spilled glue on it.
19. Easy. One part mom. One part dad. Two parts poop.
20. I'd rather have beer money.

Things to Never Say to Your Pregnant Partner . . . or Should You?

1. T
2. F
3. T
4. F
5. F
6. T
7. F
8. T
9. F
10. T
11. F
12. T
13. F
14. T
15. F
16. T
17. F

Kiss That Life Goodbye

- day drunk
- sleep late
- wild party
- silence
- privacy
- not smelling like pee
- going out
- money
- sexy time
- no vomit
- whims
- cool cars
- dry clothes
- adult things
- ninja swords
- speeding
- cursing
- seedy friends
- time alone
- full night sleep
- irresponsibility

Who's Your Baby?

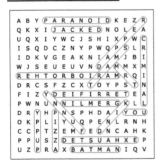

Who Will I Be?

1. Doesn't know where to find the peanut butter. Says "Ask your mother" for every question, including "How are you doing?"
2. Speaks in grumbly sighs and pained expressions.
3. Calls kids "slugger" and "champ." Talks about throwing around the ol' (whatever ball is available)
4. Dad who thinks he's humorous. No one else really does, but they're polite to him about it . . . usually.
5. Tries to use language designated for younger crowd. Uses it wrong. Puts "the" in front of everything—the Instagram, the Twitter, etc.
6. Has a story about everything that goes back to "his day."
7. To a kid, any of us. All of us.
8. Uses militant language to "get things in shipshape." Most susceptible to rude faces and hand gestures when back is turned.

Second Try, Mister

1. A
2. A
3. D
4. A
5. A
6. C
7. D
8. A
9. A
10. D
11. D

Crossing Words and Changing Bodies

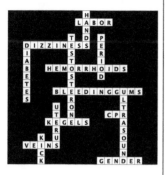

That's a Terrible Name There, Sparky

Answer:
ALL OF THEM

Hi (BLANK), I'm Dad

1. holy
2. scarecrow
3. blind
4. cemetery
5. tan
6. spill
7. nails
8. chocolate
9. scrambled
10. foneral
11. toad
12. toothpaste
13. milkshake
14. idea
15. stung

Bigger Than a Breadbox

- peach
- lemon
- rubber duck
- Beanie Baby
- soda can
- grapefruit
- coconut
- cantaloupe
- one pound coffee bag
- bread loaf
- half gallon milk
- five pounds flour
- soda liter
- sock monkey

It Does a Body Good

1. Folic acid and iron
2. Omega-3 fatty acids
3. Brain freeze
4. Giant forearms, ability to punch bullies across room
5. Amino acids
6. Calcium
7. Turn blue; turn mushroom house invisible
8. Beta-keratin
9. Reveals the Matrix
10. Protein
11. Gas
12. Monosaturated fatty acids
13. Detective abilities
14. Hydration
15. Rabbit harassment

Anazítisi: From the Greek for "Search"

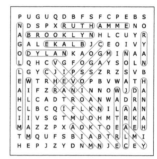

Farewell, Wall Reef

brag, below, study, real fun, listen, chin, thing, race, present, santa, dessert

Stay Away from My Baby Mama!

1. T
2. F
3. T
4. F
5. T
6. T
7. F
8. T
9. F
10. T
11. F
12. F
13. T
14. F
15. T
16. T
17. F

Scrambled Life Lessons

1. charitable
2. kindness
3. courage
4. intelligence
5. sportsmanship
6. compassion
7. strength
8. humor
9. organization
10. fitness
11. loyalty
12. trustworthiness
13. faithful
14. humility
15. perfection

Searching for a New Life

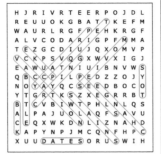

(BLANK) This

1. fool
2. pee
3. boring
4. lefts
5. leg
6. fish
7. life
8. head
9. sell
10. team
11. borrower, lender
12. better
13. free

A Tale as Old as Dad

married, lives, the best things in life are free, game of life, listen, older and wiser, young lad, bedroom, kitchen, shack, castle, kids, door, cared, teenager, mother, pal, mate, friend

Dirty Diaper, Filled Butt Pillow

1. Nummies Sequel
2. Lil' Soggy Bottom
3. Squooshy Tooshie
4. Boogz
5. Peeper Creepers
6. Premium Unleaded Baby Fuel
7. Spittle
8. Little Presents
9. Wee Wee Pads
10. Stinky Binkies
11. Little Mister/ Miss Stinker Pants
12. Baby Unplugged
13. Leaky Lil' Face
14. Teeny Slippery Fingers
15. S.S. *Floatie Doo-Doo*

What the Frig!

1. T (German: Hellfire)
2. F
3. T (French: Poop)
4. F
5. T (Amharic: "You are the fatty layer on my warm milk")
6. F
7. T (Swedish: Butthole)
8. F
9. T (Arabic: "Your butt is red!")
10. F
11. T (French: Wanker)
12. F
13. T (Japanese: "You," but in a rude way)
14. F

Grand, Father

1. Grandparent
2. Insult
3. Grandparent
4. Insult
5. Grandparent
6. Insult
7. Grandparent
8. Insult
9. Grandparent
10. Insult
11. Grandparent
12. Insult
13. Grandparent
14. Insult
15. Grandparent
16. Insult
17. Grandparent
18. Insult
19. Grandparent
20. Insult

Third Try, Mister

1. D
2. D
3. A
4. A
5. A
6. A
7. D
8. A
9. D
10. C
11. A
12. C

Baby Froop

wonderful, dangerous, fathers, bleach, shelf, accidents, sharp, laceration, open flames, smoke and fire, trouble, fire extinguisher

A Rose by Any Other Name

1. Peter Hernandez
2. Eric Bishop
3. Robyn Fenty
4. Stefani Germanotta
5. Onika Maraj
6. Christopher Cooksey
7. Aubrey Graham
8. Christopher Bridges
9. Leslie King Jr.
10. Mark Sinclair
11. Carlos Estevez
12. Margaret Hyra
13. David Jones
14. Brian Warner
15. Floyd Joy Sinclair
16. Henry Samuel
17. Clifford Smith Jr.
18. Jim Hellwig
19. Scott Thompson
20. Ferdinand Lewis Alcindor Jr.

Watch Your Language

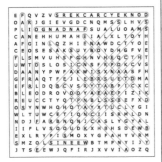

Happily Never After

1. Girl kills long-time resident. Sets out with three friends to kill her sister.
2. Inanimate objects fight. Nearly get killed by neighbor. Battle for the love of a little boy.
3. Girl gets poisoned. A group of miners keeps her in the woods. A stranger kisses her without her consent.
4. Two sisters. One has a problem with ice.
5. Residents of inner city struggle with addiction and literacy. One neighbor lives in a trash can.
6. Boy gets bullied. Reads book. Rides giant dog. Watches horse drown in mud.
7. Flying nanny encourages children to self-medicate with sugar.
8. Monster forces girl to live with him. Love story.
9. Octopus takes girl's voice. Forces her to trick sailor into marriage.
10. Old man pretends wooden doll is his son.
11. Man gives up on his dreams. Tries to kill himself on Christmas. Fails.
12. Kid watches other children die on factory tour. Enjoys songs from indentured servants.

Say This/Not That

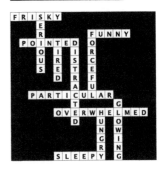

Goodbye Yedboog

- sleep
- nice clothes
- privacy
- partying
- clean home
- silence
- money
- dangerous toys
- fast cars
- crazy friends
- lazy mornings
- bar nights
- keggers
- whims
- last minute trips
- morning sex

A World Full of Bosj

actor, artist, director, dentist, educator, mayor, student, waitress, welder, teacher, pirate, parrot

Scrambled Eggs

1. fetus

2. teething
3. infant
4. womb
5. preemie
6. nipple
7. nursing
8. ultrasound
9. crying
10. formula
11. stork
12. soothe
13. rash

Nursery Rhymes Are Crazy

1. T (Three Blind Mice)
2. T (Old Mother Hubbard)
3. F
4. T (Old Woman Who Lived in a Shoe)
5. F
6. T (Jack and Jill)
7. F
8. T (Hey Diddle Diddle)
9. F
10. T (Little Miss Muffet)
11. F
12. T (Humpty Dumpty)
13. F

Falling Fast

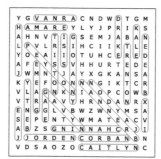

Dad Word Puzzle

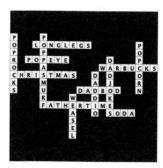

We're Having a (BLANK)!

1. delivery
2. parking
3. raising a baby
4. diapers
5. epidural
6. gelatin
7. mittens
8. heads
9. bath
10. toots
11. vomit
12. skin

You're Doing It Wrong, Honey

1. T
2. F
3. T
4. T
5. F
6. T
7. F
8. T
9. F
10. T
11. F
12. F
13. T
14. T
15. F
16. T

Put Away Your (BLANK), Dad!

1. healthy
2. one hour
3. smoke-free
4. two years
5. check-ups
6. vaccinations
7. denist
8. mistreatment
9. eats
10. age-appropriate
11. love, support

No More Tries, Mister

1. A
2. D
3. A
4. A
5. B
6. A
7. D
8. A
9. A
10. A
11. A
12. A
13. D
14. A

Safety or Fakery?

1. T
2. F
3. F
4. T
5. F
6. T
7. T
8. F
9. T
10. T
11. F
12. F
13. T
14. F
15. T
16. F

A Widdle-Piddle Wordy-Searchy

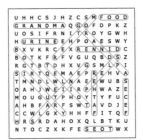

Go for It, Partner!

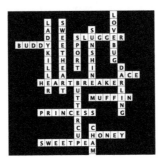

Famous Baby or Famous Monkey?

1. Baby ("Charlie Bit My Finger")
2. Monkey (Donkey Kong)
3. Baby (Maggie Simpson)
4. Monkey (Bubbles)
5. Monkey (Curious George)
6. Baby (the Olsen twins)
7. Baby (Baby Spice)
8. Monkey (Mr. Teeny)
9. Monkey (Dr. Zais)
10. Monkey (King Kong)
11. Baby (Bamm Bamm)
12. Monkey (Albert II)
13. Baby (Baby Houseman, *Dirty Dancing*)
14. Monkey (The Monkees)
15. Baby (Baby Yoda)

Searching for the Answers

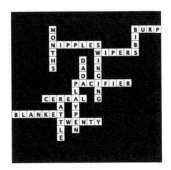

What We Say and What They Hear

1. Kneel on the kitchen counter.
2. Leave one cookie in the package.
3. Hold the dog in front of her face for two seconds, then run away with it.
4. Sit on the kitchen floor and watch us cook dinner.
5. Get finger-prints on the hallway outside the bathroom.
6. Skip your English, sci-ence, and social studies homework.
7. Toss your dirty shoes onto the carpet when you come home.
8. Make sure you wear dirty pants.
9. Sit awake in bed for three hours before someone walks by and notices you there.
10. Yell at your sister.
11. Stick that pencil in your nose.
12. Drop all your food on the floor.
13. Do it but hide it.
14. Be at a home, anybody's home, by 10 p.m.
15. Ball this up and stick it in your drawer.

Duck Logo (Good Luck)

made, aunt, begin, Rome wasn't built in a day, rooster, garbage man, swing, cried, heart, smile, face, coolest

Kids' Books

1. Girl devours cupcakes. Turns colors. Eats different food. Turns different colors. Doctor doesn't see a problem.
2. Bird demands the right to steer public transportation vehicle without a license.
3. Formal salutations to celestial bodies for some strange reason.
4. Stuffed bear talks with British accent, eats marmalade.
5. Small bug eats pieces of the book you are holding.
6. Little boy is forced to go without dinner. Hungry, he hallucinates that he's on an island with monsters.
7. Cat, naked except for a few accessories, terrorizes children home alone.
8. Baby with one crayon draws a whole world. No adult super-vision at all.
9. Dilapidated train relies on hope to get up a hill, narrowly avoiding crash and certain death for all below.

10. Annoying creature bugs other creature to eat rotten breakfast in strange locations.
11. Monster warns you not to turn pages of book. Ignore him. Teaches to ignore rules.
12. Neglected boy forced to live in a closet is sent to a school where wizards try to kill him.

Lyrical Masterpiece

- fight
- hardworking, the best you can
- soul, soul
- preacher's
- knock, knock
- dance
- coming home
- killed, head, dead
- trouble, sleep
- dances, beautiful

Scrambled Kid Culture

1. Elmo
2. Dora
3. Peppa Pig
4. Wiggles
5. Raffi
6. Mickey Mouse
7. SpongeBob SquarePants
8. Spider-Man
9. Barney
10. Thomas
11. My Little Pony
12. Buzz Lightyear
13. Hulk

Happy Holidays, Sad Wallet

1. Star Wars figure
2. Cabbage Patch Dolls
3. Transformers
4. Teddy Ruxpin
5. Nintendo
6. Teenage Mutant Ninja Turtles
7. Beanie Babies
8. Tickle Me Elmo
9. Tamagotchi
10. Furby
11. Wii
12. iPad
13. Fingerlings

Buy This, Not That

1. Y
2. Y
3. N
4. Y
5. Y
6. N
7. N
8. Y
9. N
10. Y
11. N
12. Y
13. N
14. Y
15. N
16. Y
17. N
18. Y
19. N

Secret Dad Message Incoming

Answer: QUIT DOING PUZZLES AND GO CHANGE YOUR BABY. THE WHOLE HOUSE STINKS AND WHILE YOU ARE AT IT, YOU SHOULD TAKE A SHOWER, TOO. USE SOAP. WHAT THE HELL DO YOU THINK THIS IS?

Cow El Me, Baby!

delivery, disgusting, worry, dread, process, experience, parenthood, family, together, itinerary, reevaluate, important, nothing, memory

Uncool Running

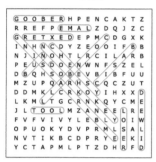

Ode to the Final Scramble

- yesterday
- trimester
- colic
- adventure
- begins
- father
- fear
- worry
- waited
- instincts
- reach
- tight
- grown
- child
- warmth
- grateful
- years
- live

Resources

Books

Caring for Your Baby and Young Child, 7th Edition: Birth to Age 5 by
     American Academy of Pediatrics and Tanya Altmann, MD, FAAP
Dad is Fat by Jim Gaffigan
Home Game: An Accidental Guide to Fatherhood by Michael Lewis
*The Baby Owner's Manual: Operating Instructions, Trouble-Shooting Tips,
     and Advice on First-Year Maintenance (Owner's and Instruction Manual)*
     by Louis Borgenicht, M.D., and Joe Borgenicht
What to Expect the First Year by Heidi Murkoff

Websites

AAP.org (American Academy of Pediatrics)
BabyCenter.com
BabyChick.com
Healthline.com
HealthyChildren.org
Parents.com
SleepFoundation.org/articles/children-and-sleep
WhatToExpect.com
WomensHealth.gov/pregnancy
ZeroToThree.org

Apps

Contraction Timer
Daddy Up
Pregnant Dad
What to Expect

References

BabyCenter. Accessed May 11, 2020. BabyCenter.com.

Centers for Disease Control and Prevention. Accessed May 11, 2020. CDC.gov.

Gabillet, Annie. "A Week-by-Week Fetus-Size Guide Based on Objects You Actually Know." PopSugar Family. June 8, 2018. PopSugar.com/family /How-Big-My-Baby-43786310.

Huggies® Diapers. Accessed May 11, 2020. Huggies.com.

Johannes, Lesley-Anne. "Covid, Corona, and 61 Other Names You Won't Believe People Actually Gave Their Kids." *Parent*. April 8, 2020. Parent24 .com/pregnant/baby-names/61-of-the-worst-names-parents-actually-gave -their-kids-20180815.

June, Laura. "How to Deliver a Baby (If You Absolutely Have To)." *Cut*. March 1, 2016. TheCut.com/2016/03/how-to-deliver-a-baby.html.

Misurelli, Anna, Elizabeth Sarah Larkin, Heather Djunga, Mark Lugris, Simon Books, Alexandra Sakellariou, Margarita Olivares, et al. "The Trusted Source for Pregnancy Info Parenting News." BabyGaga. May 11, 2020. BabyGaga.com.

Parenting Science—The Science of Child-Rearing and Child Development. ParentingScience.com.

PBC Expo Shop. PBCExpo.com.au.

SafeWise. "Child and Baby Safety Archives." Accessed May 11, 2020. SafeWise.com/blog/category/child-and-baby-safety.

Acknowledgments

Thank you to the readers of HiBlogImDad.com and all my readers through the years!

About the Author

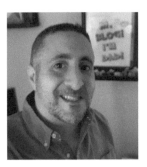 **James Guttman** is the dad behind the *Hi Blog! I'm Dad* blog and the *Hi Pod! I'm Dad* podcast, where he talks about raising his two children—a nonverbal son with autism and a nonstop verbal daughter without autism. His writing has appeared on Love What Matters, the Mighty, Yahoo Lifestyle, and Autism Speaks. You can follow him on Twitter, Instagram, or any social media @HiJamesGuttman.